Getting Research into Practice

Edited by

Collette Clifford PhD MSc RN DipN(Lond) DANS RNT ITLM

Professor of Nursing, School of Health Sciences, University of Birmingham, Birmingham, UK

Jenny Clark MSc Cert RGN RM RHV

Senior Lecturer, School of Health Sciences, University of Birmingham, Birmingham, UK

Foreword by

Alison Norman CBE HonDSc RN RM RHV DMS

Visiting Professor of Nursing, University of Staffordshire, Director of Nursing and Operations, Christie Hospital NHS Trust, Manchester, UK

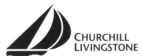
CHURCHILL
LIVINGSTONE

EDINBURGH LONDON NEW YORK OXFORD PHILADELPHIA ST LOUIS SYDNEY TORONTO 2004

CHURCHILL LIVINGSTONE
An imprint of Elsevier Limited

First published 2004

ISBN 0 443 06050 9

British Library Cataloguing in Publication Data
A catalogue record for this book is available from the British Library

Library of Congress Cataloging in Publication Data
A catalog record for this book is available from the Library of Congress

Notice
Medical knowledge is constantly changing. Standard safety precautions must be followed, but as new research and clinical experience broaden our knowledge, changes in treatment and drug therapy may become necessary or appropriate. Readers are advised to check the most current product information provided by the manufacturer of each drug to be administered to verify the recommended dose, the method and duration of administration, and contraindications. It is the responsibility of the practitioner, relying on experience and knowledge of the patient, to determine dosages and the best treatment for each individual patient. Neither the publisher nor the editors assumes any liability for any injury and/or damage to persons or property arising from this publication.

The Publisher

 your source for books, journals and multimedia in the health sciences

www.elsevierhealth.com

The
publisher's
policy is to use
**paper manufactured
from sustainable forests**

Printed in China

Contents

Contributors

Ros Carnwell BA MA PhD RGN RHV CPT CPT Cert Ed (FE)
Professor of Health and Community Research, Centre for Health and
Community Research, North East Wales Institute, Wrexham, Wales, UK

Jenny Clark MSc Cert RGN RM RHV
Senior Lecturer, School of Health Sciences, University of Birmingham,
Birmingham, UK

Collette Clifford PhD MSc RN DipN(Lond) DANS RNT ITLM
Professor of Nursing, School of Health Sciences, University of
Birmingham, Birmingham, UK

Jane Coad PhD BSc(Hons) PGDip RGN RSCN
Lecturer in Nursing, School of Health Sciences, University of
Birmingham, Birmingham, UK

Carol Dealey MA BSc(Hons) RGN RCNT
Research Fellow, Research Development Team, University Hospital
Birmingham NHS Trust, Queen Elizabeth Hospital, Birmingham, UK

Paramjit S. Gill DM MRCGP ILTM
Clinical Senior Lecturer, Department of Primary Care and General
Practice, University of Birmingham, Birmingham, UK

Joy Grech RGN RSCN
Research Nurse, PICU, Birmingham Children's Hospital NHS Trust,
Birmingham, UK

Maggie Griffiths RGN BA(Hons) MSocSci
Lecturer/Research Associate, School of Health Sciences, University of
Birmingham, Birmingham, UK

Christine Henderson MA MTD DipN RM RN
Research Fellow, School of Health Sciences (Nursing), University of
Birmingham, Birmingham, UK, and
Editor of the British Journal of Midwifery

Chris Holden RGN RSCN MSc MCRIG (City and Guild)
Nutritional Care Sister, Nutritional Care Department, Birmingham
Children's Hospital NHS Trust, Birmingham, UK

David Jones RF
Lecturer, Department of Primary Care and Population Sciences,
Royal Free and University College Medical School,
Whittington Hospital, London, UK

Liz Morgan RGN RSCN RCNT RNT DipNEd DipHSM MSc
Head of Nursing, Birmingham Children's Hospital NHS Trust,
Birmingham, UK

Peter Nolan PhD MA BEd(Hons) BA(Hons) RMN RGN DN RNT
Professor of Mental Health Nursing, School of Health, Staffordshire
University, Stafford, UK

Howard Shaw MA PhD AHSM DMS
Senior Research Manager, DHSC: Midlands & East of England,
West Midlands R&D, Government Office for the West Midlands,
Birmingham, UK

Maureen Smojkis MSc BSc(Hons) DipSN RMN
Lecturer in Counselling and Programme Coordinator, Solution-Focused
Brief Therapy, Centre for Lifelong Learning, University of Birmingham,
Birmingham, UK

Kent L. Woods MA MD ScM FRCP
Professor of Therapeutics, Division of Medicine and Therapeutics,
University of Leicester, Leicester, UK, and
Director, NHS Health Technology Assessment Programme

Pat Wrightson MSocSc BA MCSP DMS DipTP
Professor of Physiotherapy, School of Health Sciences, University of
Birmingham, Birmingham, UK

Foreword

Why is it essential that we get research into practice?

The answer can be readily adduced from healthcare history and indeed from some current experiences, both in the UK and overseas.

A hero of mine, and a pioneer of evidence-based practice over a century before the phrase was coined, is Ignaz Semmelweis (1880–1865), a physician at the Lying-In Hospital in Vienna. Semmelweis became aware of the high level of maternal mortality due to puerperal fever. It was reputed that women would beg to be allowed to have their babies in the street and then return to the hospital, such was the reputation for death by that institution. Semmelweis believed that the puerperal fever was caused by medical staff coming straight from the post mortem room to the delivery room without washing their hands. His action in introducing the simple practice of hand washing hugely reduced the mortality rate. He was, however, not honoured for this breakthrough. Experienced practitioners resented the change and, perhaps as Austrians, were adverse to taking instruction from an Hungarian.

Today, we have a different challenge in the management of sepsis. In the UK maintaining and improving standards of cleanliness has become an issue, rehearsed regularly in the press and has required Department of Health action to restore public confidence.

The inappropriate and over prescription of antibiotics (against best practice evidence) is a problem throughout the developed world. It is predicted that this might create new epidemics of 'super bugs' as destructive in our age as puerperal fever was in 19th Century Vienna.

The controversy around the combined measles, mumps and rubella vaccine provides evidence of a new problem. This is the means by which healthcare research is disseminated to the public and clinicians and the impact that it then has. The initial research paper published by Andrew Wakefield and colleagues from the Royal Free Hospital in 1998 postulated a possible link between the vaccine and rising rates of autism and bowel disease. The study was very small, looking at 12 cases only. However, its impact has been powerful. Despite an active campaign by other researchers and the Department of Health the uptake of MMR has dropped from 92.5% to 79% nationally and in some parts of London has dipped to 61%. There is now real concern about a measles epidemic that could cause death and disability.

Whatever the rights and wrongs of this issue, on the basis of published research there never has been a strong case for linkage for the administration of MMR and the development of autism and bowel disease. However, the impact on the public through the media has been profound. Professionals have appeared unable or unwilling to refute the claims and influence patients to have their children vaccinated. This possibly being due to their understanding of the weight of research evidence in support of the vaccination.

The above cases illustrate the importance of the mainstream of the profession understanding enough about research and the means of dissemination to be able to influence their own practice and the service provided by organizations.

Health practitioners also need a clear appreciation of the expectations now laid upon them. These are that care and treatment should be provided efficiently and effectively to a significantly more knowledgeable public. The availability of information through the internet and the growth of patient support and disease orientated groups has brought about a welcome shift in the balance of power between clinician and patient. The onus is now on the practitioner to be able to share information and knowledge and to demonstrate practice which is commensurate with guidance and standards freely available to a discerning public.

Increasingly this will require organizations as well as individuals to put in place the means by which evidence-based practice is the norm.

Fortunately, the Department of Health focus on clinical governance has enabled Trusts to pay proper attention to their performance in this regard. It has also empowered individuals and groups to flag needs and concerns and to have some expectation that these will be addressed.

This book provides a resource to assist the practitioner with an interest in research as well as those seeking inspiration to support their research study or research aspirations. It should also stimulate readers to take action in their own sphere of practice to bring forward the research agenda. In reflecting on our history and some current challenges it is also important to recognize how far we have come in the past 15 years within the UK.

The chapters dealing with healthcare policy, resources and organization provide an excellent background to the establishment of a national research and development programme and the impact that this has had on the service.

The importance of the coordination, prioritization and focussing of effort and resources is clear as is the improvement in managing the research agenda to maximize benefits. The need for linkage between NHS development and research may seem obvious but was not properly in place prior to the 1998 House of Lords Review of Research and Development (R&D) in the NHS.

A system of research governance mirroring clinical governance principles and massively improved dissemination and utilization. This has been through the efforts of the National Institute for Clinical Excellence, the use of health technology assessment and implementation of National Service Frameworks, leading to real progress in producing an evidence base for practice, and indeed demonstrating a service fit for purpose in the 21st Century.

For most of us the priority must be to ensure that available evidence is properly understood, introduced and bedded down in the front line of care. This text goes on to assist us with the means by which change can be brought about, essential if improvements are to be sustained and a post code lottery of care quality is to be avoided. The chapters dealing with practical experience provide a range of evidence from the individual practitioner to the evolution of a professional evidence base. Two quotes from this section struck me with particular force. 'Research into practice is much more than merely doing research projects in practice, it is about the right research being done, it is being owned by all concerned and the findings being valued and implemented', (Ch. 9, Smojkis & Nolan). In Chapter 12 we are reminded that 'Using research is not an optional extra, rather it is an intrical part of professional practice' (Clifford).

The use of research may be multi-faceted. These facets include an eagerness to receive knowledge, the ability to evaluate material critically and to have determination and willingness to embrace change on the basis of knowledge gained. Equally it may require us to be more individually active as participants in research or as a leader of research.

The achievement of a position where we can all genuinely claim to use research in practice and to have a sound evidence base to our work is dependent upon a number of effective partnerships: government and the NHS must put in place an effective and properly resourced R&D network; non-governmental independent research organizations and the NHS must work together to maintain and sustain complementary research programmes; the NHS and higher education institutions must work together to provide joint appointments and shared initiatives; and service organizations must bring forward clear research strategies, for their partners and shareholders, which set out reality and aspiration as a public means of engendering both internal and external synergy and development.

Local strategies should recognize the importance of the D in R&D and ensure the opportunity to develop research capacity and capability within the mainstream of the service as well as supporting the research effort at the leading edge. We all have a part to place in this endeavour. This book is a means of enabling readers to play their full part.

Manchester, 2004   Alison Norman

Preface

About 20 years ago the focus of healthcare research tended to be uni-disciplinary. Moreover, much of the debate and discussion was underpinned by the idea of getting healthcare practitioners to do research. There was a notion that if we increased the number of health professionals who were research active we would be able to do 'better research'. For those who thought about it there was a strong feeling that if we could address issues related to doing research, increased insights would change the way we worked and used research and develop a stronger 'research culture'. Generally, we gave little thought to the challenges facing other professional groups struggling with the same agenda. For many there was a perception that professional groups established in the university system had developed their research agenda and that other professional groups needed to 'catch up'.

At the beginning of the 21st Century we can acknowledge that both our uni-disciplinary focus and the emphasis on increasing the 'doers' was rather naïve. We certainly needed the doers but in the later years of the 20th Century we learned we needed a lot more. We learned that there were more commonalities than differences in the ways in which individual healthcare professional groups tried to get to grips with an emerging research agenda. We saw knowledge about optimal ways of doing research in healthcare increase. There was increased recognition of the importance of using the findings from high-quality research studies, focusing on cumulative research findings rather than single projects to inform clinical practice. We lived through a relocation of healthcare education for many professional groups from the health service to the higher education arena resulting in increased emphasis on research as an area of education and practice. Addressing all these issues to varying degrees we saw the growth of a national research and development strategy that was designed to develop healthcare research and support practitioners in their efforts to get research into practice.

The impact of these changes served to encourage many healthcare practitioners to think about ways in which their practice was informed by the most up-to-date research findings. At one level lack of knowledge was such that it was acknowledged that primary research was undertaken to address knowledge deficits. To do this there was undoubtedly a need to develop a cadre of high-quality researchers who could do the research to an appropriate standard. At another level, where a lot of research existed, the art of systematic review was developed to determine the implications of research findings for clinical practice. It was recognized that not only was there a need to help practitioners make sense of the findings from research evidence available, but that specialist skills were required. It is important to note that having research findings available in key areas of healthcare practice does not mean that there is a sound research available.

From an organizational perspective healthcare managers were being asked to account for research activity in their clinical areas. Staff working in higher education recognized the need and educators were busy trying to find the best ways of helping students learn about research so that they could, in due course, contribute to the research agenda. In summary, much was happening in the healthcare research world at the end of the 20th Century.

It is this range of activity that this book is about. The context is set by describing the evolution of a national research and development strategy. Consideration is then given some of the organizational issues that may impact upon clinical practitioners ability to use research in their practice. This is followed by a number of individual case studies across a range of healthcare professional groups and a variety of healthcare and education settings as the authors describe their experiences of endeavouring to impact on the research agenda.

In many respects these are the untold stories of the evolution of a national research and development strategy, the impact on the 'shop floor' in healthcare as a whole range of people contribute towards developing a strategic vision. The cases illustrate the complexity facing researchers, clinicians, managers and educators who are working to improve the use of research in their own environments. Hopefully, by bringing the range of experience together into one text alongside strategic and organizational insights, readers will be better placed to consider the issues that they may face in their own area of work as they try to develop the research agenda. In summary, it would appear that whilst strategies to develop research activity can be successfully implemented the multiple dimensions that may impact on using research in practice remain a challenge. It is hoped the lessons outlined in this book will go some way towards helping future healthcare professionals address the issue of getting research into practice.

Birmingham 2003   Collette Clifford

Acknowledgements

This book would not have been possible were it not for the efforts of a very large number of people who have worked with, collaborated or generally supported the authors of the chapters in the book. Names are too numerous to mention but you will know who you are. Thank you for helping to increase the insights and understanding of the challenges faced by those endeavouring to get research into practice in healthcare.

PART 1

Context

PART CONTENTS

1

Introduction

Collette Clifford

INTRODUCTION

This book is about research in healthcare practice. The aim in adopting a title that actively links research to practice is to demonstrate the context in which some aspects of healthcare research and development (R&D) have been developed in one country over a number of years. As will be seen in the early chapters in the book, a great deal of work has recently been undertaken to develop a framework to support knowledge development through research in healthcare. It was not so many years ago that little was known about the scope and nature of healthcare research, nor were there systems for managing and commissioning research to address priority areas of healthcare practice. Here, there are clear indications of a successful policy agenda that has supported the coordinated development of research in healthcare practice.

As the strategic drive for research management was evolving, questions began to emerge about the use of research in practice, the development arm of R&D. As will be seen in Chapter 2, it became evident that simply doing research was not enough; the challenge was to make the link between emerging research findings and healthcare practices. This resulted, in the 1990s, in the development of a new idea – 'getting research into practice'. This in turn evolved into the movement that was initially known as 'evidence-based medicine' (Sackett et al 1997), evolving in turn into 'evidence-based practice', to be more inclusive in healthcare delivery (see Chs 2 and 3).

The notion of getting research into practice was associated with the early efforts of a range of individuals to contribute to the evolving R&D agenda. As this developed, many healthcare organizations were challenged to consider the extent to which research featured in clinical practice. This in turn led to many initiatives, as staff working at local level endeavoured to contribute to the evolving research agenda.

It is this aspect of local activity that forms the middle section of this book. Interest in sharing experiences began some years ago when various contributors were working on different aspects of research in healthcare. At that time new strategies for the management of health service research were being developed and, within this, there was a move to enhance both the quality and the quantity of health service research. The challenge facing many professional staff was that new R&D strategies were being introduced into healthcare systems that, for many professional groups, had not previously had a formalized research agenda. There could be said to be a divide between the rhetoric of those who were, quite rightly, promoting high-quality research to inform healthcare practices, and the very much larger group of practitioners who were increasingly being expected to use research findings in their practice but who had little knowledge of the processes involved.

For some, this created an opportunity to learn about and explore ways of doing research in their practice within a recognized managerial framework. For others it was more challenging, as the changing expectations about using research were happening at a time when, for many, the very concept of research was new. Research as a topic had not been a traditional part of educational provision in many professional preparation programmes and was only becoming fully established as part of professional curricula at the same time as the UK National Health Service (NHS) R&D strategy was being developed (see Ch. 2). Consequently, there were a number of situations where the first step in any plan to 'get research into practice' and enhance the evidence-based healthcare agenda was to get baseline data about what staff knew about research at the outset. If staff had no knowledge of research then how could they use the emerging findings? As with any new development, this led to the uncertainties imposed by challenges and changes to traditional practices.

The accounts in this book are important in recognizing the overall impact of the NHS R&D strategy, for they demonstrate the learning that occurred at this time and the challenges faced as staff grappled with changing paradigms in healthcare delivery. While the outcome of some of the work discussed can be seen in professional journals, other aspects, such as organizational issues, cannot, since the presentation of such issues is often confined, for example, to local discussion forums. These experiences are nevertheless an important part of informing the understanding of the overall impact of implementing a strategy that focuses not only upon research but also on the development of practice based on research – i.e. some of the ways of getting research into practice.

The chapters in the book are written by a range of healthcare professionals including nurses, physiotherapists, doctors, midwives, health visitors, managers, educators and researchers working across a range of healthcare settings. This strategy was adopted to demonstrate that the challenges faced in contributing to the evolving NHS R&D agenda were not uni-professional or uni-role, or of relevance to only a limited range of care settings, but rather that common issues are faced by all healthcare professional groups, regardless of the location of their work. Readers are advised to consider this when reading the text and not to discount the experience described because it is not focused in their particular area of practice or written by someone in their own professional group. There are key principles in all chapters, relevant to all, as will be seen below.

FRAMEWORK FOR THE BOOK

The framework for this book is illustrated in Figure 1.1. This shows a number of factors that impact on research and related practice in healthcare. The first relates to *healthcare policy*, an aspect that impacts directly upon resources available and, through managerial channels, the level of organizational support committed to any changes in practice. The second group of issues relates to professional readiness for research which requires a sound *educational* base. This encompasses issues related to initial professional education, continuing professional development, and partnerships between education institutions and clinical centres to facilitate education and research developments. The third relates to the availability of *knowledge* generated through research. This can be linked to customary or traditional ways of practice that are at times hard to challenge, particularly when professional groups are convinced they are approaching care in the best way. In traditional models, knowledge is transmitted on the basis of personal experience or professional authority (Robinson & Vaughan 1992). This in turn relates to organizational readiness to embrace new knowledge as it becomes available. A final grouping of factors links *dissemination* of research to the healthcare professions and to the general public. Changing expectations accompanied by developments in technology mean that research information may reach professional groups at the same time as it reaches the general public, a relatively new phenomenon in healthcare. Each aspect will be discussed briefly below.

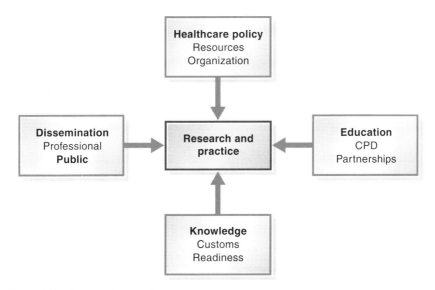

Figure 1.1 Context of research.

Healthcare policy

The starting point in this book is consideration of the model of healthcare policy that has reframed the way in which publicly funded healthcare research is managed in the UK. As will be seen in Chapters 2 and 3, coordinated efforts have made a major impact on the ways in which research is managed in healthcare.

Health policy changes have led to new ways of working and introduced a new language to healthcare management. For example, the concept of clinical governance reflects present ideology in healthcare, putting the patient or *user* of services at the heart of managerial policy (see Ch. 4). The notion of governance is now commonly referred to in wide-ranging aspects of clinical management. If care is to be delivered optimally, not only must issues related to local care organization be considered but there is also a need to consider whether the care delivered is to an optimal level based on the most up-to-date knowledge (see below).

Linked with this is the need to ensure that the staff who deliver care are adequately educated to deliver optimal care. In the context of research, this implies their having sufficient knowledge of research processes to be able to use the knowledge available. As a result, in healthcare today, we see managerial frameworks referred to as 'research governance' (Clifford 2003). While there may be much debate about the origins and influences of differing healthcare policies, from the perspective of research in practice they have made a clear difference to the ways in which publicly funded healthcare research is managed. From historical patterns in which research management was either non-existent at worst or ad hoc at best, this must be seen as a major achievement.

Resources

Clearly, resources are required to undertake healthcare activities. Resources may be defined as, for example, the funding required to pay for staff to undertake research. At another level resources may refer to the infrastructure required to undertake the research. In the case of laboratory-based research, for example, this may refer to the availability of the laboratory space necessary to do the work; for other types of research it could be, for example, the computing systems necessary to allow data to be analysed.

It is a simple fact in the modern world that if any activity is to be developed resources are required. Activities associated with health policy statements generally do have resources identified. This may mean new funds are identified; however, it is not uncommon in publicly funded activities for funding to be redirected. This pattern is evident in healthcare research strategies. As noted in Chapter 2, funding for research was previously available, but, in healthcare, use of such funds has been associated historically with hospital centres located near to universities. Such funds may have been used well, but the direction of activity towards areas of real need was not apparent. Hence the necessity to focus research on healthcare priorities noted in Chapters 2 and 3.

Organizations

The organizations through which healthcare is delivered are variable in scope and purpose, ranging from the high-technology environment of an acute hospital to the types of organization that endeavour to maintain healthcare in the community. Whatever the nature of the healthcare business, organizational support is required before any changes can be implemented. Here the link with healthcare policy is clear as, in the busy modern world, a major driver to ensure organizational support is given to any strategy is to tie it in with organizational targets. The link to resources becomes apparent as NHS organizations are now asked to identify spending on research and related activity. With the advent of an NHS R&D strategy, health service managers became accountable for research work undertaken in the locality. Accountability for resources in research is now an integral part of the research governance agenda in the NHS (see Ch. 2). It may be suggested that this was one way of stimulating organizational support in organizations that had not hitherto been involved in explicitly making commitments for research developments.

Education

The next group of factors looks at issues to do with education. In this book we can only touch the surface of the vast educational changes that have occurred in healthcare in the UK in the last 10–15 years. This has far surpassed the changes experienced in the previous 50 years of the NHS in which most healthcare professionals with a 'hands-on' role in care giving have received formal training in healthcare settings. For most professionals, with a few exceptions – for example disciplines such as medicine, dentistry and psychology – the emphasis was on skills acquisition and in general little time was spent on developing the thought processes required to take a more analytic approach to work or the critical thinking skills that underpin research.

While such a statement may be seen by many as contentious, it is important to contrast the skills-based training of many healthcare professionals with the academic training afforded by universities where the concept of research is integral to learning. Traditional healthcare education more commonly presented information to students as a series of facts to be acquired with little exploration as to how these facts had been come by. Interest in research began to expand with increased affiliation with the higher education sector in the late 1980s and early 1990s.

In this text we have endeavoured to illustrate the implications of this transition by tracking the evolution of the profession of physiotherapy. While this group is now firmly located in the university sector, it was not always so. As will be seen in Chapter 6, the transition from health service models of training to a university-based educational programme, and the impact of this in contributing to the developing research agenda in health-care, was not straightforward and involved major professional redirection. This pattern can be seen in all the healthcare professions that have made a similar transition.

Continuing professional development

The concept of continuing professional development (CPD) is integral to the educational agenda in that there is a critical need to ensure that all healthcare professions maintain the skill and competencies required to deliver health-care. In the context of research developments, however, there is another very important issue: determining how best to make up for the knowledge deficit that is a reality for many healthcare professionals who undertook professional training in old-style NHS programmes. As noted above, many of these programmes did not consider research to be an integral part of the curriculum. Hence, when policy planners began to explore ways of getting research into practice, for many qualified staff the first step in this process was meeting an educational deficit in healthcare practitioners (Clifford & Murray 2001). As the 'new' generations – that is, those healthcare professionals who have received a university-based education – begin to take leadership roles in healthcare, the challenges from a CPD perspective are not to introduce research processes but to find ways of making research accessible and meaningful and to support staff in developing the skills required to make changes in practice, should the evidence generated by research require them to do so (see Chs 4 and 5). This issue has continued, and will continue, to be a challenge (Thompson et al 2001, Bryer et al 2003).

Partnerships

The issue of partnerships has been alluded to above in the context of health-care education, with many healthcare professionals moving to the higher education sector giving universities the remit of preparing the next generations of healthcare practitioners. Early efforts in this area were considered problematic by some groups, as many thought the pendulum had swung too far away from the practically based training of the NHS towards the kind of academic preparation offered by universities (Department of Health 1999). In more recent years, clear efforts have been made to address this issue and new structures in healthcare organizations are designed to support partnership arrangements between university and healthcare systems. This addresses, at one level, issues related to educational preparation and provides ways of exploring the use of research in practice, aspects that are now an integral part of undergraduate curricula for healthcare practitioners (Clifford et al 2002).

At another level, the importance of healthcare researchers working within the university sector has been acknowledged within NHS R&D structures. Here it is noted that funding awarded to support research activity will be allocated on the basis of a number of criteria, one of which is collaborative arrangements between the NHS and the university sector. The simple reason for this is that universities are deemed to be the centres that have, overall, the greatest expertise in developing research. In encouraging such partnerships NHS planners have been working to ensure that those who undertake research in the NHS do so with the best available support and guidance (http://www.doh.gov.uk).

In some areas where there are already well-established relationships between the university and local healthcare units, such arrangements have been working well for many years. For others this has proved more challenging as new partnerships have needed to be developed, building, in many cases, new ways of working.

Knowledge

One means of generating knowledge is research, and the intention to develop the 'best' knowledge on which to base healthcare practice was a key factor in the formation of the NHS R&D agenda. Knowledge is, however, a very diverse concept that will be considered in this book from the perspective of the way in which knowledge is developed (i.e. the research approaches adopted) and also, less directly, from the point of view of issues relating to the level of individual practitioners' knowledge about research. Quite simply, if healthcare practitioners do not understand both research processes and the implications of research findings, they will not be able to make informed decisions that will impact on their practice – it will not be possible to determine whether patients are receiving the best care possible based on the most up-to-date knowledge. Thus the link between education and knowledge development is clear, for it is through education that the practitioner learns how to do research and how to critically read research findings.

One of the real challenges facing many healthcare practitioners is how best to use knowledge either when knowledge is scanty or when the knowledge available is not conclusive. Hence the need to combine difference forms of knowledge, i.e. the knowledge generated via research and the knowledge that falls into the domain of 'best known' practice. This reflects the evidence-based agenda which is discussed in more detail in Chapters 2, 3 and 4.

Customs

One of the biggest challenges facing those wishing to implement research is the acknowledged tendency for custom and traditional practices to become the norm. It is quite feasible that approaches to care that fall into the mode of 'custom and practice' may indeed be the best way of care delivery, but the challenge to healthcare practitioners today is to feel confident that their customary practice would stand up to scrutiny by research.

Most professional groups can give examples of aspects of care delivered by previous generations that have been discredited by later generations. This does not mean that previous generations were uncaring, rather it is a reflection of the time they were working in: with the knowledge available to them at that time they *thought* they were giving the best care. The same proviso will apply to the present generation in due course. We do, however, have the benefit of insight into research and recognition that just because something appears to work with our groups of patients, this does not mean it is necessarily the best way of giving that care. For this reason it is not unusual in healthcare for research to be undertaken into aspects of care that we think are best, as a means of either confirming or refuting our perceptions.

There are two challenges here. The first is to encourage practitioners to question their own practice. To do this we need to consider the second challenge, that is, how to help practitioners who have always worked in one model of care giving (i.e. custom and practice) to be open to new ways and to develop the capacity to question their practice. Commonly, while individual resistance to change must be acknowledged (see Chs 4 and 5), it is often the case that people are reluctant to change because they have never been helped to do so. Thus the link with education emerges again.

The challenge for those who do understand this is to find ways of assisting others to feel confident that research is evident in their practice, helping them to develop ways of working that challenge the customs and the ritual of traditional practice and to keep an open mind about the optimal ways of working.

Readiness

The notion of readiness applies to both individual and organizational factors and links to the issues discussed above in terms of being prepared to challenge traditional ways of working. For an environment to be responsive to research it requires commitment at both the individual and the organizational level. It will become evident in this text that individual readiness will impact upon the capacity of organizations to respond to health policy directives. But it is not a simple process. If the individuals within organizations do not understand research, or if they feel resistant to it, this will impact upon organizational readiness. It is for this reason that several contributors to this book set out to determine to what extent individual practitioners could contribute to the research agenda (see Chs 7, 8 and 9).

As indicated above, organizational readiness can be associated with healthcare policy and associated resources. Information now readily available on the Department of Health website (http://www.doh.gov.uk) shows that there is diverse research activity across a variety of healthcare settings. The link with resources is evident in that some very active research-orientated health units may have multi-million pound research budgets identified. In contrast, others have relatively small sums allocated. Here the resource issue can be clearly related to the skill base of staff, since if there are only a limited number of staff available who understand research then it is unlikely that a given unit will have a big research budget. From another perspective it can be seen that often those centres with large research budgets are those that have long-standing association with staff in university posts who have had sufficient training to lead research programmes. It is also worth noting that there is a difference between 'readiness' and ability, a factor that is very well illustrated in Chapter 11. Those responsible for leading organizational R&D agendas need to consider these diverse aspects when implementing their research governance systems.

Dissemination

There is a simple formula that can be applied to research, as illustrated in Figure 1.2. Here the steps of the process can be tracked from the initial idea, through to data collection and analysis by whichever method is seen as appropriate (see below), leading to the preparation of a research report. Depending upon the outcome, the cyclical process may be repeated. This occurs, for example, if the answers to the initial questions are not clear enough (see methodology section below).

Generally speaking, at the end of a research project, a research report is presented. In recent years there has been an increased emphasis on finding ways to make this information readily available to healthcare staff to inform their practice. It is self-evident that if research findings are not disseminated then the work cannot be used to inform the knowledge base of practice. In short the work is wasted, for there is little point in undertaking research if the findings are not made available. Historically the most common way of publishing research work has been in professional research journals. Those that are seen as the most credit-worthy are those that carry peer review status – that is, these journals do not publish the outcome of research unless it has first been subjected to critical review by professional peers. In theory, this enables the publishers to establish how sound the research is as well as to identify any aspects of the research that are unclear prior to their appearance in the public domain.

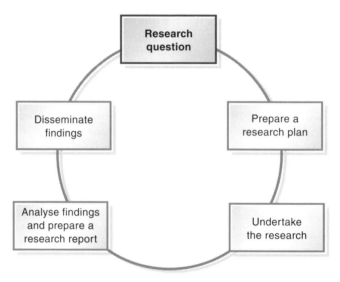

Figure 1.2 The research cycle.

Despite the massive and steadily increasing number of published health journals, a number of topics remain for which the answers as to the best ways of providing care are not clear. For this reason, as will be seen in Chapters 3 and 4, new ways of making information available to healthcare practitioners have been explored. They include making the outcome of publicly funded research readily available to all those who need it, commonly via websites. This means that members of the general public, commonly referred to as healthcare users, can access information as quickly as healthcare professions, since most dissemination websites can be readily accessed by all (see below). This is an important point as it represents a major shift from healthcare practices of years gone by when professional groups had a monopoly on health-related information. As will be seen in Chapter 2, this exclusivity is no longer acceptable, but the wide availability of evidence from research means that healthcare practitioners are likely to be working with patient or client groups who are much better informed than earlier generations, another critical reason to ensure that healthcare practitioners are equally well informed.

Availability of research to professional groups

All healthcare professionals should be using relevant research findings to inform their practice. This may seem self-evident but it is an aspect that creates challenges for healthcare planners. For example, as indicated above, in order to be able to use research effectively, staff need to have sufficient understanding to read research critically and make judgements about it to determine whether it is sufficiently robust to inform any practice development or changes. This may seem an obvious and easily achievable goal but it should be noted that although insights into research methodology are now an integral part of educational programmes for healthcare professionals, this was not always the case. Thus the knowledge level required for this level of activity may be limited. Moreover, even this simple observation shows a degree of naivety for it is most unlikely today that a single research study would stand alone as an argument for practice change. It is more likely that cumulative evidence, drawing upon the output from a number of projects, would be required. This involves the ability to undertake critical review of a range of research methods involved in researching a particular area of practice and using the collective input from a number of projects to draw conclusions about the 'optimal approach' to care. Such work is undertaken under a process known as 'systematic review', commonly by people who are specialists in this aspect of research. It is acknowledged that what healthcare practitioners need is access to information provided as the result of such reviews rather than expecting each individual practitioner to undertake individual reviews. Information of this nature is now readily available to all via a range of web-based resources (discussed in Chs 2, 3 and 4).

There is, however, one problem here that should be noted. Because much of the research into aspects of healthcare is relatively recent, systematic reviews may come to the conclusion that there is lack of sufficient evidence to recommend 'best' practice. The practitioner who has attempted to find out information may then be faced with uncertainty; however, with the system available under the NHS R&D umbrella, he or she is able to inform the NHS of the need to undertake research in that aspect of care (see Ch. 3).

Public dissemination

One critical factor that should be noted is that dissemination as an art form has moved away from just seeking the best ways to inform healthcare professionals and now also includes consideration of how best to inform the general public about the status of the most up-to-date evidence. The advent and increasing sophistication of information sources through the world wide web means that the general public can access information as quickly as the healthcare professions. This has implications for health professions, who are no longer custodians of unique knowledge, but again it raises the need for practitioners to be well informed on the implications of information that may be widely available to the general public.

This does create new challenges, for there is a need to help people discern between sound research evidence and customary practice that can be readily drawn out on a web search for the best ways to manage a specific health problem. Many self-help groups offer websites on which they present what they feel to be the 'best' treatment options for particular health problems. Not all of this advice is grounded in sound research knowledge. This situation can challenge healthcare practitioners and again reinforces the need for all to be able to distinguish between research knowledge and custom and practices when working with patients.

Linked with this, concepts such as 'transparency' and 'openness' are commonly cited as desirable in societies such as that in the UK. It is not uncommon to have wide public debate on the outcome of research work and indeed for the general public to exercise their right to challenge research outcomes. This has been seen recently, for example in the UK where there has been open debate about the risks of children receiving the combined measles, mumps and rubella (MMR) vaccine. Here, differing interpretations of research findings have influenced the way in which parents view the vaccination programme for children (http://www.nelh.nhs.uk/hth/mmr.asp). A user perspective is now an integral part of the NHS R&D strategy just as it is central to the overall health service policy (see Ch. 2).

A WORD ABOUT RESEARCH METHODOLOGY

The word 'research' implies a cyclical process with the notion that we search out information and then, in the light of our new knowledge, search again, i.e. re-search. The ways in which we can undertake that research are varied and there are a number of different methods which can be used. As will be seen in Chapter 5, research is a vehicle by which we develop knowledge but the ways in which we can do that are numerous. In this book, brief descriptions of aspects of research methodology are given where relevant but readers wishing for more detail should consult the many available texts that describe and critique different research methods.

The consideration of knowledge development through research, regardless of method, is, however, worthy of further note here. The aim of research is to inform healthcare practice in a positive way by directing our actions or, sometimes, by stopping us undertaking actions that may prove futile. In some cases, however, research activity fails to provide sufficient evidence to recommend any specific action and, in so doing, raises further questions for research. This is often linked to issues related to the research design or the methodology adopted. There are many challenges to researchers seeking to set up the 'perfect' study in the real world of healthcare today.

For this reason, research is in reality often less simple than the formula illustrated in Figure 1.2, which shows a cyclical process with a defined beginning and end. Sometimes the circle is completed, but a more common sequence of events is the one demonstrated in Figure 1.3. Researchers start with a question, undertake the research activity and draw their conclusions. Even for quite small-scale activity, this can be a complex process in healthcare, as illustrated in Chapter 10. If the conclusions stand up to critical

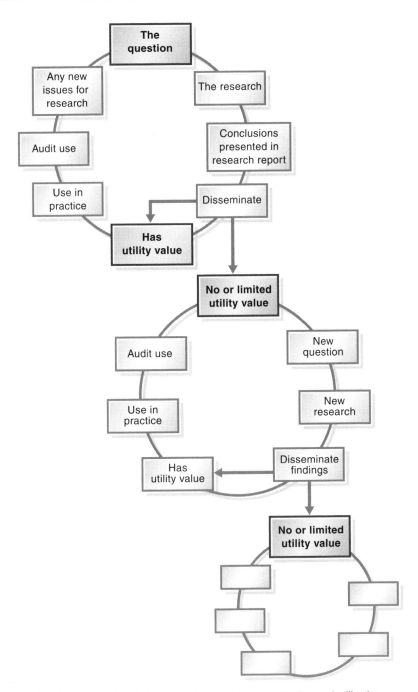

Figure 1.3   The research activity cycle – from idea to dissemination and utilization.

scrutiny following dissemination there may be a case for informing actions in healthcare. Healthcare managers will then be likely to examine the impact of the research through the usual auditing processes to determine the impact of the new approaches on care. This process may generate further questions for research.

If, as is commonly the case, conclusions are not clearly drawn, or if following dissemination healthcare managers do not find the research convincing enough to change care, perhaps because of limitations in the research design (see Ch. 11), the cycle starts again. Space does not permit an unlimited number of iterations of this process in Figure 1.3, but the number of cycles will vary depending upon the initial research question and the research design.

In summary, the number of iterations in any attempt to explore aspects of healthcare through research studies will be dependant on many factors, as outlined above. They include aspects related to methodology and, in addition, existing knowledge, healthcare policy, education, public expectations, professional development, managerial support, resources, organizational readiness and individual motivation.

FORMAT OF THE BOOK

This book is presented in three parts. The first part focuses on the context in which research is undertaken and includes strategic and management issues. This includes consideration of the context of healthcare delivery, issues related to change management, and some points to consider when proposing to undertake research in practice.

The second section offers a series of practical experiences. It begins with an account of an experience of moving the professional education of a professional group from the NHS to the university sector. This is followed by a series of accounts of efforts to influence the research agenda in a range of practice settings. The chapters focus upon a range of issues, from attempts to gather baseline data to inform the development needs of groups or practitioners to experiences of doing research in practice settings.

To set the scene, most chapters begin with a brief, discipline-specific, historical account of research developments. Hopefully this will help readers to draw comparisons with their own professional group. There are, overall, more similarities than dissimilarities.

The final chapter is a reflection on the accounts given in the book in which the implications for future developments are drawn out.

SUMMARY AND CONCLUSION

This introductory chapter has given an overview of the text that will follow. It is noted at the outset that this is not a 'how to do it' research text;

rather, it focuses on a number of broader issues ranging from strategic planning for healthcare research to local endeavours to develop, disseminate and use research in clinical practice. Consequently the perspectives vary from managerial and organizational issues to a variety of personal experiences of research activity in healthcare

This wide range of perspectives enables consideration of the policies and directives that can influence the ways in which research is developed and some of the challenges faced by healthcare professionals who want to contribute in some way to the research agenda. In offering the collection of experiences presented it is hoped that greater understanding of the complexities of developing and implementing a research and development agenda will be evident. It is acknowledged that another set of contributions could bring a different perspective. Nevertheless the underlying issues will be helpful in trying to understand the overall processes, which are relevant to all. As will be seen in Chapter 12, many lessons have been learned as a result of efforts to respond to a national research strategy.

REFERENCES

Bryer R M, Jose Closs S, Baum G et al 2003 The Yorkshire BARRIERS project: diagnostic analysis of barriers to research utilisation. International Journal of Nursing Studies 40: 73–84

Clifford C 2003 Research governance – the challenge. Nursing Times Research 8(1): 7–16

Clifford C, Murray S 2001 A pre and post test evaluation of a project designed to facilitate the development of research in practice in a hospital setting. Journal of Advanced Nursing 36(5): 685–695

Clifford C, Murray S, Kelly S 2002 Clinical effectiveness, education and healthcare practitioners. Learning and Teaching in the Professions 1(1): 6–21

Department of Health 1999 Making a difference. Stationery Office, London

Robinson K, Vaughan B 1992 Knowledge for nursing practice. Butterworth-Heinemann, London

Sackett D L, Strauss S E, Richardson W S, Rosenberg W, Haynes R B 1997 Evidence based medicine and how to teach it. Churchill Livingstone, Edinburgh (2nd edn 2000)

Thompson C, McCaughan D, Cullum N, Sheldon T, Thompson D, Mulhall A 2001 Nurses' use of research information in clinical decision making: a descriptive and analytic study. University of York Report. Presented to the NHS R&D programme in evaluating methods to promote the implementation of R&D. University of York, York

2

Research in healthcare: establishing a national research and development programme

Howard Shaw   Collette Clifford

> **Editors' comment**
>
> *This chapter gives an overview of a national strategy for developing research in healthcare. It considers strategic development, evidence-based practice, consumer expectations, disseminating research and the present agenda for managing the quality of research in healthcare today.*

INTRODUCTION

This chapter will explore a number of aspects related to the management of research in healthcare. The major focus will be on developments in England because to endeavour to explain the differences across the various parts of the UK might only serve to confuse. The general principles can be applied across all areas and the details acquired by looking at the relevant health department websites. In general, the National Health Service (NHS) in Scotland, Wales and Northern Ireland has followed the same path as the NHS in England, sometimes leading and sometimes following. The problems faced by all have much in common and there has been much sharing of experience.

This overview of one nation's developments will start with some historical observations. We then consider the development of the Department of Health NHS research and development (R&D) strategy and management, the issues of R&D prioritization, and standard setting in R&D, including consumer issues. R&D will be related to the development of evidence-based healthcare. The chapter will conclude with a discussion of some unresolved issues.

HISTORICAL PERSPECTIVE

There has been a long tradition of research into healthcare, particularly with a clinical focus, in the main university teaching hospital centres in the UK, dating from the 19th century. The National Health Service Act (1946), which established the NHS, recognized the linkage between healthcare, education and training, and research. It laid a specific duty on the secretary of state to provide facilities for teaching and research within the NHS to honour the partnership with the Ministry (later Department) of Education, to support the education of medical students. This established an early research base for medicine in general, focusing particularly on the activities of doctors since of all the healthcare professions doctors were the most active in the field of research. At that time little or no provision was made for other healthcare professions to be research-active as most staff were non-graduates and had a training base located in the NHS, in contrast to doctors who had been university-based. This meant that research was not part of the education agenda of these other professions (see Ch. 6).

The government has had a longstanding role in funding medical research through the establishment of the Medical Research Council (MRC) in 1913 as a response to the then major public health problem of tuberculosis. It is noteworthy that, at its establishment, the government made it clear that doctors rather than politicians would determine the MRC's research priorities. From the 1960s, regional health authorities (RHAs) funded small-scale R&D to encourage newly appointed consultants to develop their R&D interests as well as funding research fellowships particularly for junior doctors. The Department of Health has had a policy research programme for many years, primarily to answer questions of particular importance to ministers. A number of medical charities, such as the British Heart Foundation and many hospital trust funds donated locally, have for many years funded much medical R&D.

The seminal 1988 House of Lords review of R&D in the NHS (House of Lords Select Committee on Science and Technology 1988) convinced the government of the day that a more coordinated approach to R&D in the NHS was essential. It argued for the appointment of a national R&D director and for the RHAs to appoint regional R&D directors. Following the appointment of the first national director, Professor Michael Peckham, and the publication of the first 'Strategy for research in health' (Department of Health 1991), a national R&D programme was established to address major areas of R&D needed by the NHS, complemented by regional R&D programmes.

At this time many of the major undergraduate and postgraduate teaching hospitals, particularly in London, implicitly used substantial exchequer revenue funds to support R&D activity. These funds were originally grouped with funds to support undergraduate and postgraduate medical education. With the introduction of the recommendations of the resource allocation working party (RAWP) (Department of Health 1976) the service increment for teaching (SIFT) was identified formally. In the later 1980s the research component was recognized and the budget renamed 'service increment for teaching and research' (SIFTR) but the R&D component was never quantified.

The advent of the Thatcher market reforms to the NHS in the 1990s meant that both these funds needed to be identified and managed in a more explicit way. In 1994 a committee chaired by Professor Anthony Culyer from York University advised ministers (Department of Health 1994) that these funds should be brought into a single national funding stream subsequently known as 'Budget 1' or, colloquially, 'Culyer funds'. As a result an exercise was to be carried out to ensure that in the framework of the SIFTR funds noted above, there was no cross subsidization between R&D and patient care or vice versa.

This exercise was carried out in 1996/7, drawing on 1995/6 financial returns from clinical units. Opinions have always been divided both within and outside the Department of Health about exactly how accurately this, the so-called 'Culyer declaration', was done. However, it is acknowledged that this was a complex exercise since it was the first time that declarations of funding activity had been separated in this way. This work remains important as there was some movement of funds when the original Culyer (Budget 1) budgets for NHS organizations were set following a major national bidding exercise but little overall change since that time.

Allocation of funds at local clinical level did raise one important issue: the need for local management structures for research. One highly significant change that followed the costing exercise was the appointment of R&D directors and managers at clinical unit level, hospitals and community units managed under the umbrella title of 'NHS trusts'. These post-holders were given the responsibility to manage the funds on behalf of the various NHS bodies. This reflected a growing recognition that NHS trusts had to take responsibility for the R&D taking place within their boundaries and manage this activity accordingly.

In the early years of the NHS R&D programme there was a widespread belief that R&D should expand – indeed, ministers at one time committed themselves to NHS R&D spending 2% of the NHS vote, the part of public expenditure devoted to the NHS. This led many to argue for R&D becoming a more dispersed activity both geographically and throughout all professions. However, progress on this front was linked with the relative power of regional as opposed to national R&D.

As an example, the Mant Report on R&D in primary care (Department of Health 1997a) advocated a substantial increase in expenditure in this particular area. The simple rationale for this was that research in this sector was under-funded compared with that in the acute care sector (i.e. hospitals). This led to ministers making a specific commitment to double R&D investment over 5 years in primary care. In addition many RHAs invested in R&D support units to facilitate the development of R&D in areas where there had been little activity before. For example, in the south-west region, a region-wide network was established between 1993 and 1995 (Hamilton 1997).

During 1996 the RHAs were abolished and their successor bodies, the regional offices of the NHS Executive of the Department of Health fulfilled some of their functions. Eight of these were established in England. However, this structure was relatively short-lived and the policy document

Shifting the Balance of Power (Department of Health 2001d) established new managerial structures as a result of changing government policies. This established four directorates of health and social care of the Department of Health to replace the NHS Executive regional offices. This included the establishment of primary care trusts (PCTs) to lead the organization of care in the community and to take the lead in commissioning care from the local acute and non-acute (mainly secondary care) NHS trust providers. These PCTs would be performance-managed, as would NHS trusts, by the new strategic health authorities (SHAs) as the 'local headquarters of the NHS'. This new structure meant that the days of any Department of Health 'outposts', for example the four directorates of health and social care (DHSC), which included R&D, outside the two administrative centres of London and Leeds, were numbered. The closure of DHSCs in 2003 (Department of Health 2003b) effectively marked the end of regional R&D and the possibility of any radical dispersal of R&D activity.

Within these changing structures, for reasons that are not entirely clear, though some progress was made towards allocating the 2% of the NHS vote towards R&D activity, latterly the percentage of the NHS vote spent on R&D has actually fallen. This probably reflects changing government priorities and the relative importance different secretaries of state attach to NHS R&D.

The strength of the regional R&D offices was that they tried to respond quickly to local pressures for R&D and tried to link R&D with other NHS activity, such as postgraduate education in healthcare, as well as attempting to be very creative in their use of R&D. Their weakness was that there was a great deal of duplicated effort between the different regions. This is important, given that one of the key factors promoting R&D activity in the NHS at the outset was the need to streamline activities (Peckham 1991). On reflection it may be acknowledged that mistakes were made and there was too much micro-management of projects. However, this can be seen in the context of new organizations finding their way, and it should be noted the NHS research programme was shaped for the better by the mixed economy of national and regional R&D activity.

PRIORITIES FOR HEALTHCARE RESEARCH

In 1988, the House of Lords strategic overview of NHS research activity (House of Lords Select Committee on Science and Technology 1988) identified an uncoordinated approach to the identification of research priorities. It was perhaps a fair assessment to say that in common with research in other fields, healthcare research was more often driven by the sustained interests and curiosity of the researcher – 'investigator driven' – rather than having any strategic focus on healthcare needs – 'needs led'.

Though many leaders of the key healthcare professions saw the development of an intellectual base to healthcare as being central to its development, in general within the NHS hierarchy, R&D historically was seen as something slightly marginal. It was regarded as something that, for example, bright or intellectually curious doctors and other health scientists did, rather than an activity contributing to the growth of the NHS or providing answers to the best way to deliver the wider healthcare agenda. This is not to say that investigator driven research was not important nor that it did not make a significant intellectual contribution, but rather the lack of strategic direction and coordination meant that more resources could have focused on the main health problems faced by the NHS. It is a central question for all research funders to decide what research to fund. There are two dilemmas: the balance between investigator driven/needs led research and that between high-quality, relatively unimportant research or lower-quality relatively important research. The evidence, such as it is (Fears & Poste 1998), suggests that a 50/50 split between investigator driven and needs led research is the best way to proceed. However, funding low-quality research is never worthwhile as little notice is taken of it because it does not provide a reliable evidence base for clinical decision-making.

For the first time, the advent of the NHS R&D strategic framework (Department of Health 1993) gave the opportunity to address these issues and align the main health problems faced by the nation to the research agenda. This was important, for there was little evidence to indicate whether research being undertaken in healthcare reflected the real needs of the health services or whether agendas were being driven by the personal interests of researchers. The way in which research was commissioned is fundamental to this.

Commissioning research

In essence, the commissioning process involves an organization that is willing to fund research deciding, by some means, the type of R&D they want to fund and the questions to which they want answers. They then use some process, usually competitive, to find the best research team to provide the answer. This can be compared with investigator led research, where it is the researcher or research team who decide what they think may be worthy of research and then make an application for funding to a relevant funding body.

In both commissioned R&D and investigator led R&D, it is almost universal practice, at least among the funders with large R&D budgets, to use independent expert peer review to assess not only the quality of the research protocol but also the track record of the research team – to determine if they are capable of carrying out the research proposed to a high standard – and the generalizability of the likely result. Hence the shorthand of 'three Ps and a G' to R&D quality: *protocol* driven, *peer* reviewed, *publishable* and *generalizable*. In the context of this text the notion of whether a piece of research is publishable is critical, for it would not be possible for research to be used if others did not know about it. The notion of generalizability is particularly associated with research undertaken within the positivist research paradigm, such as projects utilizing experimental approaches (see methodology section below).

Peer review is a process that calls upon experts in the field to make judgments on the aspects outlined above. It is worth noting that the peer review process has often been criticized for its partiality and its capricious nature. However, its use continues in the absence of anything better. The move to all R&D being peer reviewed which could be deduced from a casual reading of the Research Governance Framework (RGF) (Department of Health 2001c) (see below) may force a reassessment of this model due to the shortage of experts making its widespread use impracticable.

In deciding how to use NHS R&D funds, the national R&D director also has to consider which other funders are providing funding, particularly since some funders favour particular types of R&D, in order to ensure more complete coverage. In the early years of the NHS R&D programme, for example, it was felt that quantitative research was favoured over qualitative and that R&D into aspects of clinical practice was favoured over R&D into service organization and management. As will be seen below, without any great attention being focused on it, subtly the NHS R&D programme, particularly through the service delivery and organization (SDO) programme, has embraced these differing R&D approaches.

Determining priorities

Typically, the criteria used for priority setting were:

- Burden of disease – the extent of population morbidity and population mortality related to the disease
- Cost of the disease to the NHS and to society generally
- Availability of suitable methodologies to tackle the question
- Availability of research teams to tackle the question
- Likelihood of an answer being produced
- Impact of the answer
- Cost of the project both to the research funder and to the NHS.

These criteria conflict with each other when applied to individual areas, and various techniques such as Delphi techniques (a means of gaining consensus) were used as pragmatic ways to rank priorities in some kind of relative order. As familiarity with the process and difficulties emerged two particular techniques became part of established practice: the use of 'vignettes' and the review before actual commissioning. The 'vignette' technique, developed particularly by the health technology assessment (HTA) programme (see Ch. 3), involved getting a brief description of the problem and possible solutions to narrow down exactly what question needed to be answered. At the same time this narrowing builds support for the really important questions among the body charged with the actual commissioning.

Focusing activity

An important aspect of commissioning research is the avoidance of duplication and ensuring that any new knowledge complements existing knowledge. It is therefore common to check for the existence of a systematic review in the Cochrane Library (2003), or if no systematic review exists, to commission such a review before proceeding to commission new projects. In this way new research explicitly builds on the existing knowledge base and complements it. The NHS R&D programme specifically aided this process by devoting significant sums in the early 1990s to supporting the Cochrane Library, and indeed the Cochrane Library owes its current established status in part to NHS R&D support in its initial stages.

The introduction of the NHS R&D strategy highlighted the need to focus research on the recognized national priorities in healthcare, for example cancer, mental health, dental, cardiovascular (CVD), mother and child health, physical and complex disabilities and primary and secondary care interface. This meant research was to be based on need for knowledge – needs led activity. Following the first wave of national R&D programmes, there were calls for other thematic national programmes to be established, for example on ethnic health, but no further thematic programmes were established.

This model subtly favoured needs led research by progressively phasing out all unrestricted opportunities for researchers to pursue their own individual interests using national NHS R&D programme funds, unless of course they reflected NHS priority areas. This did not mean that such work had to stop as other funders continued to respond to unsolicited requests for investigator driven R&D proposals. Overall, the national calls for research proposals for NHS research did often actually represent a nice compromise between investigator driven and NHS needs led research by allowing researchers to bid to pursue their own ideas within the broad framework set by the commissioning teams.

Over the years the evolution of the NHS R&D strategy, alongside NHS priority setting, has led to an increasing alignment of research priorities with healthcare priorities. When the first wave of national thematic R&D programmes were coming to an end, the national director of R&D, Sir John Pattison, decided not to pursue thematic programmes. Instead he decided to continue with the three widely ranging programmes: the HTA programme (see Ch. 3), the SDO programme, and the new and emerging technologies programme (NEAT). The SDO programme was to address complex issues about service organization and delivery across the whole range of NHS activity. The NEAT programme is designed to bridge the development gap between proof of concept and the generalizable application. This structure offered a framework in which all the NHS research needs could, in theory at least, be met.

To ensure appropriate coverage of thematic areas identified as national ministerial priorities in the *NHS Plan* (Department of Health 2000a), the national director of R&D introduced the concept of 'portfolio directors' in the fields of mental health, cancer, older people, primary care, coronary heart disease, children, and diabetes. None of these had specific budgets to spend, but though these directors did rather different tasks, essentially their core purpose was to promote R&D irrespective of the actual funder, to ensure a reasonable coverage of R&D consistent with NHS needs.

In the early years of the new millennium this means that those areas of healthcare that cause the government and the nation most concern are the areas that would be seen as priorities for the NHS R&D agenda. A series of national service frameworks (NSFs) (Department of Health 1998) have set standards of care for specific healthcare problems and indicate areas for research activity. By 2003 this included cancer, paediatric intensive care, mental health, coronary heart disease, older people with diabetes, renal, children's care and long-term conditions, focusing upon neurological conditions, to follow. In an ideal world all the NSFs would have been fully informed by all the relevant R&D and the knowledge gaps used to set the R&D agenda for the next few years. However, things rarely work out that neatly, the R&D often does not exist, and there is too much urgency to produce the NSF to adequately review the R&D.

Also, in many fields there are too many R&D funders who wish to set their own agendas and keeping R&D decision-makers in touch with the needs of clinical staff is not easy. Nonetheless, a comprehensive review of the R&D behind *The Healthier Nation* demonstrated how many of the NSF recommendations are evidence-based (Centre for Review and Dissemination 2000). In addition, one of the early successes of the portfolio director approach was the grouping of the main cancer charities with the Department of Health and the MRC into the National Cancer Research Institute.

MANAGING THE AGENDA

In terms of the Budget 1 framework outlined above, there are three aspects to the management of the NHS R&D programme: what is done at national level, at regional level, and by NHS trusts. Depending upon the prevailing managerial structures, the way in which this has been carried out has been a variable over time and across organizations. The first wave of national R&D programmes was managed by staff at regional level with each region focusing on a priority area; for example, the northern regional staff managed the mental health programme. Later, however, the programmes were contracted out to university staff; for example the HTA programme (see Ch. 3) is now managed on a day-to-day basis by staff employed at the University of Southampton. To progress the Mant targets (Department of Health 1997a) in primary care, national fellowships were established on a national competitive basis. Department of Health staff initially managed the actual programme but following *Shifting the Balance of Power* (Department of Health 2001d) the programme management will be contracted out via a Strategic Health Authority.

Working with the university sector

As noted in Chapter 1, many skilled research staff are located in the university sector and a key feature of later NHS R&D strategy (Department of Health 2000b) was to find ways of capitalizing upon this resource to support the evolving research agenda. This was done in several ways. For example, recognizing the specific challenges of increasing research capacity in the primary care sector, many regions invested in local programmes to interest primary care staff in pursuing their R&D ideas. This was supported by mechanisms to involve local universities in the provision of an R&D infrastructure to help staff new to research to develop R&D proposals in primary care. They also invested in their local universities to get them to provide support across the board for clinical practitioners in their R&D endeavours (for example the Trent Institute and the Birmingham Clinical Trials Unit). These units provided specialist support to clinical staff developing research.

A central feature of the new PNF programmes (see later) was the presence of an academic partner in all substantial programmes, indeed it is one of the core criteria (Department of Health 2001a). One of the consequences of the Alder Hey inquiry (Department of Health 2001b), which reported upon bad practices in research, was the establishment of the Follett committee to advise the secretaries of state for health and education about the management of clinical academics (Department for Education and Skills 2001). Among the problems identified at Alder Hey was the question of who was really responsible for the actions of clinical academics who were effectively employed by two bodies, an NHS trust and a university. The Follett committee recommended dual accountability backed by joint appraisal and formal agreements between NHS bodies and universities to ensure explicit joint policies were in place in keeping with a similar requirement in the RGF.

Pressure within the university sector from the Higher Education Funding Council for England (HEFCE) over the research assessment exercise (RAE) has lead most universities to seek to explore new ways of managing research activity (Higher Education Research Opportunities 2003). In healthcare research, this is very dependent upon the active support of the university's NHS partners. These two initiatives have made closer working between the NHS and university R&D management essential.

Linking research with NHS developments

While some national projects became embroiled in national politics (such as the abortive attempt to establish a major national multi-centre trial for beta interferon for multiple sclerosis), some regions were remarkably fleet of foot in, for example, establishing a series of projects to support the introduction of clinical governance in the NHS. Some regions tried to commission projects that met local needs, though many of these also had national significance. For example, the West Midlands rise in emergency admissions project (Bagust et al 1999) played a significant part in the evidence for the national bed inquiry set up by the secretary of state in 1999.

The scale of regional R&D activity has been in relative and absolute decline for some years and staffing has been reduced as a consequence to reflect this. These trends illustrate the pressure on regional, and latterly central, civil service staff numbers resulting in only those tasks that need to be done by civil servants being retained within the civil service and all others being contracted out, assuming they continued. In addition, they illustrate an inexorable centralization of decisions to national level consistent with the core belief that R&D is an élite activity carried out by specialists for the benefit of the whole of the NHS.

Management of R&D in trusts initially had a major financial focus but the advent of research governance (see Ch. 1 and below) raised the profile of trust R&D management as trusts now had to formally approve all R&D taking place in their organizations. Furthermore the introduction of the priorities and needs funding (PNF) stream forced trust R&D management to take a more active role by formally structuring their R&D into strong programmes or risk losing the funds allocated for research. It also emphasized the need for universities and NHS trusts to work closely together on their R&D activities.

Just as the overall development of primary care R&D has lagged behind secondary care R&D, so research governance (see Ch. 1 and below) in primary care has lagged behind that in secondary care. However, in 2003/4 a network of specialist PCT research governance and management was established to ensure all PCTs were able to discharge their statutory duties under the RGF which included approval of all R&D done by independent practitioners, quintessentially general medical practitioners (Department of Health 2002).

Following the establishment in 2002 of SHAs as the local headquarters of the NHS with major performance management roles, the management of research governance will be transferred to SHAs in 2004/5, a move that could foreshadow a greater involvement for SHAs in R&D as the Department of Health role in R&D management is reduced (Department of Health 2001d).

Overall, all these changes show how, in most areas, R&D is now to be positively managed, and no longer allowed to take place without control or management involvement. If a longer-term detached view is taken, it can be seen that the management of R&D is steadily moving further into the mainstream as well as becoming actually more concentrated and less diffuse in its distribution.

RESEARCH GOVERNANCE

Traditionally R&D was felt to be activity which did not need a great deal of formal regulation which, it was felt, would stifle the creativity inherent in the research process. Over time the number and range of regulations has steadily increased, witness the increasing concern of the MRC and the General Medical Council (GMC) about the need for precise standards to lay down for all professional staff doing clinical R&D. Two inquiries have fundamentally changed the government's view. The first was the Alder Hey inquiry (Department of Health 2001b), which concerned retained organs and tissues from post-mortem examinations of children. The second was the Griffiths inquiry into R&D at North Staffordshire Hospital (Department of Health 2000d). It could be argued that the common theme between both inquiries was that many patients and their relatives, on realizing how they had been affected by this research, felt that the essential bond of trust between them and the healthcare professionals had been broken.

The government's response was to issue an RGF that would regulate the conduct of R&D done under the terms of reference of the Secretary of State for Health and Social Care. It placed a clear duty on the chief executive to ensure that all R&D within the NHS body complied with these standards. The new breed of R&D directors in NHS trusts effectively discharged this duty and managers were appointed following the Culyer reforms discussed above.

This development of research governance paralleled the development of clinical governance, 'A First Class NHS' (Department of Health 1998), following the Kennedy inquiry into events at the Bristol Children's Hospital (Bristol Royal Infirmary Inquiry 2001). A new duty was specifically laid on the chief executive for the quality of the clinical care in his or her trust, as well as the need for explicit standards of clinical care, and a new external inspection body was established, the Commission for Health Improvement (CHI), changed in 2003 to the Commission for Health Audit and Inspection (CHAI) (Department of Health 2001c). The RGF has had a major impact in raising the standards of research conduct as it has been progressively applied across both secondary and, latterly, primary care R&D.

EU Directive 2001 (European Union 2001), though it technically only applies to clinical trials involving medicinal products, takes this a stage further. It is to be applied to the UK from 2004 onwards and will, for example, affect the way in which research ethics committees are managed as it sets precise timetables for their consideration of R&D proposals and defines much more streamlined mechanisms for ethical approval of research.

METHODOLOGY ISSUES

It is appropriate to touch briefly upon the methodological debates that have taken place during the development and implementation of the NHS R&D strategy over the past decade. These led at both national and local level to many challenges of methodological bias that were perceived by some healthcare professions as advantaging some professions over others as well as favouring some types of R&D over others. For example, debate raged over the relative value of quantitative and qualitative methods. In essence, one camp argued the likely improvements in healthcare were, by and large relatively small, and thus only by having precisely defined questions and large clinical trials to gain the necessary data to iron out inherent fluctuations could any real progress be made. This was the large-scale randomized trial school of Collins and colleagues (Collins et al 1996), who relied upon the scientific method beloved of physical science.

The qualitative school argued that the real world was not that simple and could never be so. They sought to follow the approaches of social science where the development of empirical theory followed careful observation. They emphasized the holistic nature of healthcare and the complex interplay of physical, psychological and societal forces that could never be reduced to a large simple trial. They argued that as much effort should be put into deciding what quantitative research was done as into the research itself, because quantitative methods tended to produce a very precise answer to a limited question. However, this answer was very often only one of a whole series of questions faced by the average healthcare practitioner. There was a feeling that clinical trials answered the questions that trials could answer, which were not necessarily the most pressing ones. Different healthcare professions had different research traditions and felt more at ease with different methodologies.

These debates did not go unnoticed and much effort was put into examining different ways of approaching research in healthcare. Much of this work was commissioned through the HTA programme, and the subsequent report on qualitative research designs in healthcare (Murphy et al 1998) was a major breakthrough in making the case for diversity in approach to healthcare research. The impact of such reviews were noted and the nature of the research commissioned within the NHS R&D programme changed over time from a reliance on quantitative methods, ideally in the form of a randomized control trial (RCT), to using qualitative methods where appropriate. Qualitative methods have been found to be especially useful when the area under scrutiny is not well described. In so doing it is acknowledged that they may also have a value in identifying possible questions that could be the subject of future RCTs as they try to map out the whole system as well as offering useful insights into possible implementation strategies.

DISSEMINATION AND UTILIZATION OF RESEARCH

As the new breed of R&D directors became established and insights into the research process in healthcare developed, the focus of activity began to change, particularly at regional level, as they began to realize a number of somewhat unpalatable facts.

When the NHS R&D programme started out, R&D directors saw their prime aim as being to fund high-quality R&D to provide the answers they felt the service needed and wanted. However, they soon began to see how the timetable for the R&D process was at variance with timescales set by NHS management. Managers wanted answers far quicker than R&D could produce them. They also realized that adding new knowledge was not in itself always enough. Although there were by no means answers to all the questions available from the R&D knowledge base (the research literature), it became evident that much knowledge was simply not being used, and when it was used there was an enormous time lag between results appearing in the peer reviewed journals, in text-books and in use in everyday clinical practice, for example the seminal paper on the use of thrombolytic agents for blood clotting (Antman et al 1992).

This led to the various 'getting research into practice' initiatives (Dunning et al 1998) as well as initiatives such as the West Midlands aggressive research intelligence facility (ARIF 2003) to assist health authorities and latterly PCTs in their use of R&D findings for their decision-making. It also contributed to the recognition of the need to facilitate healthcare practitioners' access to knowledge via, for example, the National Electronic Library for Health (Turner et al 2002, National Electronic Library for Health 2003).

Regional R&D directors were under great pressure to use their budgets to finance development and the greater direct utilization of R&D findings through critical appraisal training. The national response was for R&D to withdraw over time into a more focused and narrower concern for knowledge production. The field of development was taken up by the new NHS Modernization Agency when it was established in 2000 (Department of Health 2003a). In addition, workforce development confederations, the NHS bodies responsible for funding education in the NHS (Department of Health 2001d), have played an increasing role in funding various in-service training initiatives to address some of these needs.

Notwithstanding this, NHS R&D always write into their R&D contracts that all R&D must be published and have established the National Research Register (NRR) as a readily accessible means for R&D staff and clinicians to find out what R&D is taking place prior to its publication (National Research Register 2003).

EVIDENCE-BASED PRACTICE

Many studies of evidence supporting healthcare interventions in use have shown that not all are justified by high-quality research; some are simply the product of accumulated clinical wisdom derived from years of experience and some are actually of no proven value or even harmful.

In every generation of healthcare practitioners there have been practices commonly in use that were subsequently shown to be ineffective or harmful. Typical estimates of the percentage split between practices for which there is evidence, those for which there is no evidence, and those for which there is evidence against vary, but have been of the order of 60% with evidence, 30% no evidence, 10% evidence against (Ellis et al 1995, Gill & Dowell 1996, Sackett et al 2000). It would be wrong to be unduly critical of this situation as medical practice has developed over a long period of time and there are major difficulties in applying pure scientific method to clinical practice. Scientific method, simply put, involves observing a situation, proposing a theory to explain it, and then devising experiments to confirm or refute the theory. Frequently in such experiments great efforts are made to make as many factors constant as possible in order to determine the influence of the remaining factors on each other. Scientific method also assumes that the observer of the experiment does not interact with the subject, i.e. different observers, assuming they repeated the experiment in exactly the same way, would observe the same conclusion. A classic example of the application of scientific method was Louis Pasteur's experiment to show that airborne bacteria cause fermentation (Dubos 1976). There are a whole range of reasons why this approach cannot readily be applied to clinical situations but the gold standard of the RCT is perhaps the closest approximation. However, even the most basic consideration of a simple clinical situation shows the limitations of this approach and the well-known placebo and Hawthorne effects (Mayo 1949) demonstrates this nicely.

The knowledge that many established clinical practices are not evidence-based and also that many research-based practices are not always used in routine practice led Sackett and others to develop the concept of evidence-based medicine, later more widely referred to as evidence-based practice (EBP). He argued that all practitioners should use the latest knowledge as a basis of their practice and seek continually to review their practice, as new evidence became available (Sackett et al 2000).

The narrow concept of EBP can be broadened by use of the model illustrated in Figure 2.1.

This model argues that in making decisions all human beings weigh in their minds knowledge derived at the time, both explicit and implicit, knowledge of past events and their own experience, and then set these against their value system in order to interpret the information and synthesize it into a possible course of action. Sackett et al (2000) argue that to these essential

Influences on behaviour

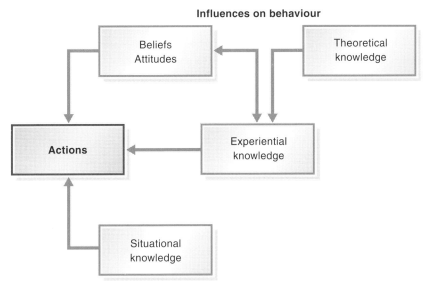

Figure 2.1   Influences on behaviour.

subjective sets of information should be added objective research evidence – evidence derived from experiments done by others. This is the force of the EBP approach.

Various studies have shown that unless people apply some mental consideration to research evidence it has very little impact, even though the facts may be known. For example, two groups of GPs were given information about the value of prescribing antibodies for viral infection. One of the groups then attended a discussion group to debate the strength of the evidence. Data were then collected to assess the impact of supplying this knowledge to GPs against a control population who were not given the materials. Only the prescribing behaviour of the GPs who discussed the evidence showed a significant change (Lagerlov et al 2000).

To illustrate the model, a GP seeing a patient with a problem of excessive drinking would wish to take a full history to determine the extent of the patient's drinking habits (explicit knowledge) as well as observing their general demeanour in the consultation (implicit information) and would review that against his or her previous experience of treating such patients. Inevitably, the GP's beliefs about alcoholism, its causes and effects, will feature in the decision-making process. EBP would argue that the doctor should also refer to externally produced knowledge about any potential intervention, for example dosage, side-effects of any drug therapy, as well as being aware of the research evidence about the treatment of patients with drinking problems.

As the work of the R&D directorate began to impact on healthcare research it became increasingly obvious that one of the major challenges to any healthcare system was not just producing the research but also finding a way to help healthcare practitioners to use the relevant findings in practice. In other words, moving from a research driven model of activity to one in which the development role – the 'D' in R&D – was fully acknowledged.

The emergence in the UK of the EBP movement paralleled developments internationally, for example in Canada and the USA. This was necessary, as it was increasingly obvious that research findings of single projects were often insufficient to inform changes to healthcare practice. Moreover, for every project promoting one line of care the discerning reviewer may have been able to identify several others with an alternative view. Consequently new terms emerged in the R&D language. This included the concept of meta-analysis. Meta-analysis is where the results from several similar studies are added together to give additional statistical significance to the conclusions (Smith & Chalmers 2001, Cochrane Library 2003). It uses sophisticated statistical techniques to review a series of research studies to determine the collective findings. Linked with this, the art of the 'systematic review' – the critical appraisal of all the research evidence on a given subject – was introduced. During this time the work of Sackett et al (2000) was influential in developing the concept of evidence-based healthcare in England. The concept brought together some of the prevailing ideologies including the need for sound research evidence, consideration of the cost of healthcare provision (i.e. drawing upon the health economics issue noted above) and the relatively new concept of patient choices (see below). It should be noted that within this framework, where research evidence was not available the recommendation was to use the 'best evidence' available but to be alert to the potential weakness in so doing and to be prepared to change if need be.

This movement informed the development of the National Institute for Clinical Excellence (NICE) (Department of Health 1995b, NICE 2003). Details of these can be found via the government website (http://www.doh.gov.uk/). The work of NICE parallels that in other centres internationally where governments worldwide have sought to introduce a fourth hurdle, that of cost-effectiveness and sometimes total cost to the healthcare system, to the existing three hurdles drugs have to pass to be licensed, namely efficacy/safety/dosage. The NICE committee considers these issues in appraising research evidence. These appraisals could include research commissioned specifically for NICE but more frequently involve synthesizing research produced by both academic and commercial research teams, including those funded by NHS R&D groups. Guidelines for practice within the NHS are produced and recommended to practitioners. Health service managers are now required to take note of these recommendations, a factor that does challenge traditional practice in which the preferences and experience of clinicians rather than any sound evidence has informed the care delivered. While there is much to commend this approach, it is worth noting that the work of NICE is not without controversy as sometimes clinicians' and users' belief in the value of specific treatments is stronger than the research evidence. This has at times generated much public debate (e.g. Dillon et al 2001, Watts 2002), which demonstrates the way in which healthcare systems are moving away from being professionally dominated systems – many healthcare users today either are very well informed or have the means to become very well informed about healthcare delivery (Muir Gray 2002).

ROLE OF CONSUMERS IN HEALTHCARE RESEARCH

Historically, much medicine was practised using a paternalistic model where the doctor was assumed to be all-knowing and all-powerful and able to command the confidence of passive patients who would simply comply with the doctor's instructions. In transactional analysis the doctor/patient relationship could be described in simple parent–child terms (Berne 1961, 1968). Under this model there was really no need for the patient to be given very much information and it was deemed unlikely that patients would seek further knowledge either from the doctor or externally. This approach could be described as 'Trust me, I'm a doctor'.

This approach in clinical practice has come under severe pressure in favour of a partnership, or adult–adult in transitional analysis terms, model (Berne 1961, 1968). In this paradigm, the doctor and patient see each other as working together to use the resources both have to solve the particular problem, sharing the information they both have. It recognizes that just as doctors will seek information from a traditional source such as a library, so patients may seek information from the Internet. This approach views patients as active sentient beings who have choices to exercise and are not merely passive partners in care (Muir Gray 2002).

This change of approach in clinical practice has had its impact on research such that the whole NHS R&D programme has sought actively to involve consumers – indeed, it is one aspect of the RGF (Department of Health 2001c). The Department of Health established the Consumers in Healthcare R&D programme specifically to take this forward (Department of Health 1999). They have explored various ways to involve consumers in all aspects of the research process from priority setting through selection of research team, project execution and implementation. Many researchers have been reluctant to accept the active involvement of consumers in R&D, arguing that R&D is a skilled expert activity. Thus, they argue that if consumers are to be constructive participants in the research process they need to be trained appropriately in how research works and given training in research methodologies. There is a danger of producing a 'catch 22' situation here in that consumers cannot make a suitable contribution to R&D because they are not trained and knowledgeable but once trained they have disqualified themselves as they are now no longer representative of consumers. This paradox should not be taken too seriously, and in fact there is much evidence to suggest that consumers do bring different perspectives to R&D and that better R&D is produced as a result. There is also some evidence that different R&D is produced as well.

Others, more cynically, might argue that some researchers were simply reluctant to cede to consumers any of their power over what they regard as 'their research'. A close scrutiny of the causes of the problems at North Staffordshire that led to the Griffiths Report (Department of Health 2000d) and those at Bristol (Bristol Royal Infirmary Inquiry 2001) with regard to the cardiac surgery and at Alder Hey (Department of Health 2001b) shows that a common theme in all these situations was that the medical profession paid insufficient attention to the rights of patients and their carers. Indeed it could be said that if more care had been given to the way things were done through the active involvement of users and carers these tragedies might not have happened.

Typical evidence that active involvement of consumers produces better R&D is that recruitment to trials has been shown to be enhanced when typical patients are fully informed about all aspects of the trial and are given the opportunity to make a major impact on the content of patient information leaflets. In terms of different R&D, when, for example, orthopaedic surgeons and patients with knee problems were asked about R&D priorities, then the surgeons argued for R&D into different surgical intervention whereas patients argued for R&D into ways to cope with reduced mobility caused by having a knee problem and not for orthopaedic solutions to the knee problem. In a slightly different context, politicians assumed, when drafting the 2001 EU Directive (European Union 2001), that patients would be reluctant to be involved in clinical trials when they were likely to have little personal positive benefit. In fact, when such potential trial patients were asked they were quite prepared to become involved.

These and other examples illustrate that clinicians cannot be representative of consumer interests; they have quite different perspectives and value systems.

All the excellent reasons to involve consumers in research notwithstanding, the practical problems are real and substantial, and individual researchers need to find ways to achieve this consumer involvement. It is, however, neither easy nor simple!

UNRESOLVED ISSUES

At the time of writing, the Department of Health/NHS R&D programme consists of the two components: PNF and support for science (SfS) (see Department of Health 2001a).

Essentially the own account part – i.e. that part of Budget 1 (see above) going to NHS bodies – has been put with the former Budget 2 to form PNF. That part of Budget 1 going to NHS bodies that supports financially the costs in the NHS of external grant-funded R&D has all been put into the new SfS budget. In 2003/4 these budgets were effectively part of one allocation to NHS bodies who could vire funds between the two parts at their own discretion. After 2004/5 it is highly likely that the two budgets will be quite separate.

The central question facing any R&D funder remains the question of what R&D to fund – a constant challenge with no simple answer. The main objectives of the NHS R&D programme are funding R&D relevant to the NHS, in particular any that other funders will not fund, the PNF programme, and supporting the costs of the MRC and medical charities in the NHS, SfS.

The PNF programme is split into centrally managed national programmes plus that managed by NHS bodies, the successor to the Culyer Budget 1 funding (Department of Health 2001a) (see above). The national PNF activity consists principally of the HTA, SDO and NEAT, plus other initiatives reflecting ministerial priorities, such as the National Cancer Research Network (NCRN). The Department of Health is encouraging NHS bodies to formulate their PNF funded R&D into coherent programmes of R&D with the underlying assumption that only strong programmes will be funded in the future. This inevitable concentration of R&D mirrors the actions of the Higher Education Funding Council for England's (HEFCE 2003a) actions in promoting excellence in university-based R&D by selectively funding only those units deemed to be of high quality. The unresolved question for the Department of Health is which NHS PNF programmes to invest in and which to dis-invest in and on what basis. With regard to SfS, the Department of Health is actively encouraging NHS bodies to recruit more patients into high quality national clinical trials, viz. the NRCN initiative; the question is how to fund this new activity in a simple way when the costs vary between trials and between NHS bodies.

Since the original Culyer declaration of 1995/6, relatively little money has moved around the NHS as ministers have believed that to do so would destabilize many NHS bodies. There is much anecdotal evidence that in different parts of the NHS significant cross-subsidization between R&D and patient service takes place. However, this position becomes progressively less and less tenable as the R&D moves around universities producing cost pressures in different NHS bodies. In addition, as the introduction of the financial flows model of funding NHS activity in NHS trusts by PCTs is progressively introduced over the years up to 2005/6, a fundamental rebasing of costs to ensure that R&D income and expenditure are in balance will be necessary. At the same time education and training activity has to be rebased so that the three potential income streams to all NHS providers are in balance. This far-reaching work will force the abandonment of the previous reluctance to move R&D funds around the NHS.

To complete the picture of the difficult choices facing the national R&D director and incidentally HEFCE, the government is committed to the expansion of undergraduate medical education involving establishing some six new medical schools in existing universities. These universities are arguing that they need extra HEFCE and NHS funds to establish R&D activity to complement their teaching activity, as occurs in all other medical schools. This also needs to be considered from the perspective of other healthcare professionals' education being located in the university sector (see Ch. 6) and the concerns expressed nationally about the need to support groups that have not traditionally led the research agenda to be able to do so in the future (HEFCE 2003a, 2003b; HERO 2003). How this will be financed is not clear. At the time of writing the government is actively considering concentrating R&D activity into a relatively small number of existing universities, a policy that could leave these new schools being part of a teaching-only higher education sector (HEFCE 2003a, 2003b). This has profound implications not only for these institutions but also for medical and other professional education.

SUMMARY AND CONCLUSION

This chapter has given a historical overview of one national R&D strategy for healthcare. It has endeavoured to track the development of the national system and the factors that have impacted upon it. In so doing consideration has been given to changing government policy and the way in which changing healthcare organizations and their structures have impacted upon the management of this national initiative.

The clear focus on developing the research agenda at the outset was noted, but in due course it was realized that this would have little value unless ways to use research better were developed in healthcare delivery. It was this shift into a consideration of ways to use research in practice that has informed many of the chapters in this book and so this chapter has relevance to all the work reported.

In conclusion, it is interesting to note that at the time of going to press, the way in which research is managed at local, regional and national levels has undergone major change but, in the intervening years, the NHS R&D strategy has had major impact on the way in which health service research generally has developed, on the fact that it is now an explicit part of heathcare practice and, importantly, on the ways in which research findings are disseminated to both practitioners and the general public.

REFERENCES

Aggressive Research Intelligence Facility (ARIF) 2003 University of Birmingham. http://www.bham.ac.uk/arif/

Antman E M, Lau J, Kupelnick B, Mosteller F, Chalmers T C 1992 A comparison of results of meta-analyses of RCTs. Journal of the American Medical Association 268(2): 240–248

Bagust A, Place M, Posnett J W 1999 Dynamics of bed use in accommodating emergency admissions: stochastic simulation model. British Medical Journal 319(7203): 155–158

Berne E 1961 Transactional analysis in psychoanalysis. Evergreen Books, London

Berne E 1968 Games people play. Penguin, Harmondsworth

Bristol Royal Infirmary Inquiry (BRII) 2001 Report of the public inquiry into children's heart surgery at the Bristol Royal Infirmary, 1984–1995. Stationery Office, London

Centre for Review and Dissemination (CRD) 2000 Contributors to the Cochrane and Campbell collaboration: evidence from systematic reviews of research relevant to implementing the wider public health agenda. NHS Centre for Review and Dissemination. http://www.york.ac.uk/inst/crd/wph.htm [August 2000]

Cochrane Library 2003 Update Software, Oxford. http://www.update-software.com/Cochrane/default.htm

Collins R, Peto R, Gray R, Parish S 1996 Large scale randomised evidence: trials and interviews. In: Weatherall D J, Ledingham J G G, Warrell D A (eds) Oxford textbook of medicine, 3rd edn. Oxford University Press, Oxford, pp. 21–32

Department for Education and Skills 2001 A review of appraisal, disciplinary and reporting arrangements for senior NHS and university staff with academic and clinical duties [Follett Report]. HMSO, London

Department of Health 1991 Research for Health September. HMSO, London

Department of Health 1993 Research for Health June. HMSO, London

Department of Health 1994 Supporting research and development in the NHS [Culyer Report]. HMSO, London

Department of Health 1995a Report of the NHS health technology assessment programme. HMSO, London

Department of Health 1995b Methods to promote the implementation of research findings in the NHS. HMSO, London

Department of Health 1996 The new funding systems for research and development in the NHS: an outline. HMSO, London

Department of Health 1997a National working group on R&D in primary care [Mant Report]. HMSO, London

Department of Health 1997b The new NHS: modern and dependable. HMSO, London

Department of Health 1998 A first class service – quality in the new NHS. HSC 1998/113. HMSO, London

Department of Health 1999 Involvement works: second report of standing group of users in NHS research. NHSE/HMSO, London

Department of Health 2000a The national plan for the NHS. HMSO, London

Department of Health 2000b Research and development for a first class service – R&D funding in the new NHS. Department of Health website http://www.doh.gov.uk/

Department of Health 2000d The report of a review of the research framework of the North Staffordshire Hospitals NHS Trust [Griffiths Report]. http://www.doh.gov.uk/wmro/northstaffs.htm

Department of Health 2001a NHS priorities and needs: R&D funding, a position statement. www.doh.gov.uk/research

Department of Health 2001b Royal Liverpool Children's Hospital inquiry report [Alder Hey Report]. Department of Health/Retained Organs Commission, London

Department of Health 2001c Research governance framework. HMSO London. Department of Health website http://www.doh.gov.uk/research/rd3/nhsrandd/rgimpplan.htm

Department of Health 2001d Shifting the balance of power. Department of Health website http://www.doh.gov.uk/

Department of Health 2002 Department of Health website http://www.doh.gov.uk/

Department of Health 2003a Modernisation agency. Department of Health website
http://www.doh.gov.uk/

Department of Health 2003b Departmental report CM 904. HMSO, London

Department of Health and Social Security 1976 Resource Allocation Working Party.
HMSO, London

Dillon A, Gibbs T G, Riley T, Sheldon T A 2001 NICE and the coverage of Relenza by the
NHS. Milbank Memorial Fund, New York

Dubos R 1976 Louis Pasteur. Scribner, New York

Dunning M, Gilbert D 1998 Research evidence and improved practice. Nursing Times 94(21):
59–60

Ellis J, Mulligan I, Rowe J, Sackett D L 1995 Inpatient general medicine is evidence based.
A-Team, Nuffield Department of Clinical Medicine. Lancet 346(8972): 407–410

European Union 2001 EU Directive 2001/20/EC on good clinical practice in clinical trials.
European Union, Brussels

Fears S, Poste G 1998 Radicalism, rationalising or rationing: what does the UK want from
research in the science base and health service? Annual SmithKline Beecham Science
Policy Symposium, 5 October, London

Gill P, Dowell A C 1996 British Medical Journal 312: 9–821

Hamilton R 1997 R&D support units: a model for encouraging health service research. Poster
presentation at the 2nd International Conference. Scientific Basis of Health Services,
October 1997, Amsterdam

Higher Education Funding Council For England (HEFCE) 2003a HEFCE Strategic Plan,
2003–08. www.hefce.ac.uk/pubs/hefce/2003/03_35.htm

Higher Education Funding Council For England (HEFCE) 2003b Joint funding bodies.
Review of research assessment

Higher Education Research Opportunities (HERO) 2003 Higher education research
opportunities in the UK. http://www.hero.ac.uk/rae/

House of Lords Select Committee on Science and Technology 1988 Priorities in medical
research. HMSO, London

Lagerlov P, Loeb M, Andrew M, Hjortdahl P 2000 Improving doctors prescribing behaviour
through reflection on guidelines and prescription feedback: a RCT. Quality in Health Care
9(3): 159–165

Mayo E 1949 The social problems of an industrial civilization. Routledge, London [reprinted
in: Pugh D S 1997 Organization theory: selected readings. Penguin, London]

Muir Gray J A 2002 The resourceful patient. Rosetta Press, Oxford, eRosetta
[http://www.resourcefulpatient.org/]

Murphy E, Dingwall R, Greatbach D, Parker S, Watson P 1998 Qualitative research methods
in health technology assessment. Health Technology Assessment 2(16)

National Electronic Library for Health 2003. http://www.nelh.nhs.uk

National Health Service Act 1946. HMSO, London

National Research Register 2003 Update Software, Oxford. http://www.update-software.com/
national/

NICE 2003 National Institute for Clinical Excellence, London [MidCity Place, 71 High
Holborn WC1V 6NA]

Peckham M 1991 Research and development for the NHS. Lancet 338: 367–371

Sackett D L, Strauss S E, Richardson W S, Rosenberg W, Haynes R B 2000 Evidence based
medicine and how to teach it, 2nd edn. Churchill Livingstone, Edinburgh

Smith R, Chalmers I 2001 Britain's gift: a 'Medline' of synthesised evidence. British Medical
Journal 323(7327): 1437–1438

Turner A, Fraser V, Muir Gray J A, Toth B 2002 A first class knowledge service: developing
the National Electronic Library for Health. Health Information and Libraries Journal 19(3):
133–145

Watts G 2002 Pharmaceutical industry guide. Health Service Journal 112(Suppl. 1)

3

Developing a research programme to meet a national agenda

Kent L. Woods

Editors' comment

This chapter gives a comprehensive account of a research programme in healthcare. It demonstrates that careful planning and coordination can result in a well-focused programme that meets the needs of people requiring healthcare today. The success of this programme in providing much needed evidence for healthcare delivery is impressive. Moreover, the ready access of research reports through websites means that, unlike in earlier times when research was only available through esoteric journals, an ideology of making research available to all who want access has been achieved. Such systems are essential to those who want to be sure that their practices are research-based.

INTRODUCTION

The National Health Service (NHS) health technology assessment (HTA) programme was established in 1993 as one of the early initiatives of the NHS research and development (R&D) strategy, of which it remains the largest research commissioning body. It currently invests £10 million per year on commissioned primary research (mainly randomized clinical trials) and secondary research (systematic reviews) (Department of Health 2002). Unlike the nine topic-focused commissioning programmes set up at about the same time – for example, those in mental health and in coronary heart disease and stroke – it was planned as an open-ended rather than a time-limited enterprise. It has therefore evolved over a decade to meet the changing research and organizational requirements of the NHS. This chapter considers:

- The scope and characteristics of HTA
- The central role of HTA in an evidence-based healthcare system
- How the NHS HTA programme operates
- The links required to make research available to decision-makers in the NHS.

These themes will be illustrated by examples relating to evolving research questions with large implications for the NHS. Reference will also be made to the interconnections which have been made with bodies set up to deliver the objectives of the NHS plan. Chief among these is the National Institute for Clinical Excellence (NICE) (Department of Health 1998). The development of these organizational links has given greater clarity to the contributions of research and of policy development (broadly defined) to individual patient care.

WHAT IS HTA?

Health technology assessment (HTA) is the branch of applied science which assembles the evidence on the effectiveness, cost-effectiveness and broader impact of health technologies. The term 'health technology' is cumbersome and open to misinterpretation – it is not confined to high technology as popularly understood, but includes all interventions used for diagnosis, treatment and rehabilitation of disease. That scope is extremely wide. It includes, for example:

- Drugs
- Laboratory diagnostic tests
- Screening tests
- Imaging
- Psychological treatments
- Surgical procedures
- Devices.

It would not, however, cover issues concerning the delivery and organization of healthcare which are now catered for by a separate programme, the NHS service delivery and organization programme.

The descriptive term HTA has persisted despite its limitations because it has now been adopted internationally and because there is no simpler term which can unambiguously describe the wide scope of the field. Nevertheless, the publicly funded HTA agencies which have rapidly been established around the world have interpreted their roles in slightly different ways. Some of these differences reflect the diversity of healthcare systems within which they operate. One feature of the NHS HTA programme which distinguishes it from most others is that it commissions not only secondary research of existing evidence (systematic reviews) but also primary research – usually a randomized control trial (RCT) – in areas where the evidence is inadequate for the needs of decision-makers. The NHS HTA programme currently has a portfolio of over 70 RCTs. Primary research is costly and carries an investment risk. It typically takes several years to complete. The return on investment may be poor, if the research results are negative. However, there are some key questions in healthcare which cannot be answered by systematic review of the existing evidence and which are unlikely to attract research funding from commercial sources. In such circumstances, it is in the public interest that well-designed primary studies should be supported.

Characteristics of primary HTA research

Although in principle the choice of research design for primary research in HTA is not restricted to randomized control trials, in practice this is the preferred approach because of the scope it offers for unbiased comparisons between one intervention and alternatives (or no treatment if there is not an accepted standard intervention). Such research typically has the following features:

- It considers the effectiveness of the intervention(s) in patient groups and under conditions which are as close as possible to routine practice.
- The outcomes of interest for judging effectiveness are patient-focused clinical end points (such as mortality, morbidity, or quality of life), rather than surrogate end points (such as blood pressure change) which are not easily interpretable in terms of clinical utility.
- Data are gathered to support health economic analysis, so that cost-effectiveness can be estimated as well as effectiveness.
- A multidisciplinary research team is needed in order to bring the required range of knowledge and skills to the project.

Trials in this area are therefore usually more complex to design and perform than might be the case with a conventional trial of a new drug, for example. The need to measure clinically relevant end points also tends to prolong the study duration until sufficient data have accrued. It is not unusual to examine several facets of treatment within the same trial, in order better to understand the contributions of various elements of a 'treatment package'. This approach stands in contrast to the reductionist approach of much therapeutic research, whereby the concern is with a single component of treatment studied in a narrowly defined patient group. The latter design choices may increase the internal validity (freedom from bias) of the study but at the cost of reducing its external validity (generalizability).

HTA trials in consequence tend to be complex, protracted and expensive to perform. Properly done, however, they should yield results which can easily be translated into the circumstances of routine care.

Systematic reviews in HTA

It is often the case that several studies have been carried out to examine the effectiveness of a particular health technology. They may vary in details of design and also in their quality and statistical power, yet each have something to contribute to our understanding of the technology. An important means of putting such a body of evidence at the disposal of decision-makers is the systematic review (Sutton et al 1998).

The essential feature of a systematic review is that it assembles the available evidence on the selected topic using systematic and explicit criteria.

This serves to minimize bias arising from the selective use of the evidence. In principle it also makes the review reproducible, though in practice it is not possible entirely to eliminate individual judgment in the selection and synthesis of evidence considered relevant. A systematic review may optionally include meta-analysis, a statistical technique to derive a valid pooled estimate of treatment effect from several independent studies.

The HTA programme has commissioned systematic reviews on a wide range of technologies, for example:

- Devices, e.g. inhalers (Brocklebank et al 2001)
- Therapeutic areas, e.g. management of dyspepsia (Delaney et al 2000) or atopic eczema (Hoare et al 2000)
- Behaviour change relevant to health, e.g. breastfeeding (Fairbank et al 2000)
- Diagnostics and screening tests, e.g. ultrasound in pregnancy (Bricker et al 2000), testing for the human papilloma virus in cervical screening (Cuzick et al 1999) or alternative strategies to detect fragile X syndrome (Pembrey et al 2001)
- Methodological issues in HTA, e.g. how to monitor surgical outcomes (Bruce et al 2001) or how to apply Bayesian statistical techniques (Spiegelhalter et al 2000).

Such work has two broad applications. Firstly, it enables decision-makers to reach judgements on the use of a technology with the benefit of a comprehensive and unbiased summary of evidence at a point in time ('decision-maker' here includes patients, health professionals and those who commission and manage health services). The second role is to identify key gaps in current knowledge. This is of value to another group of decision-makers: those who plan or commission further research on the same topic. Research funding organizations such as the Medical Research Council now recognize the importance of basing decisions about future research on a comprehensive synthesis of what is already known. The HTA programme itself, in developing the evidence base on a particular topic, has often first commissioned a systematic review and used it explicitly to develop the brief for commissioning primary research. Such an approach is particularly helpful when the implications of a new technology for healthcare are complex; all facets will need to be considered in deciding which are the critical pieces of missing evidence.

Technology assessment reports

A full systematic review of an established health technology is a lengthy piece of work for a group of researchers. Certain core disciplines will need to be represented: information science, medical statistics, health economics. In addition, clinical topic experts and public health specialists are likely to be required. For a new health technology, however, the existing evidence base will almost certainly be smaller and there will be greater urgency for the review to be available to the NHS. Since 1999 the HTA programme has directly commissioned technology assessment reports (TARs) from designated academic units able to offer the generic skills outlined above. TARs are pieces of independent academic research, carried out to a carefully agreed methodology and protocol, typically within 6 months of the commission being placed. Examples will be given below.

THE CENTRAL ROLE OF HTA IN AN EVIDENCE-BASED HEALTHCARE SYSTEM

Assessment, as has been described above, is a branch of applied science. If its results are to be used in the development of healthcare policy, a second element must be added – *appraisal*. It will be apparent that a range of factors must be taken into account when the findings of science (which by definition are generalizable) are being considered in a specific context. The evidence itself does not usually dictate what should actually be done in particular circumstances. Appraisal is an exercise of judgement which will include, in addition to the best available evidence on the effectiveness and cost-effectiveness of the technologies, such factors as acceptability, feasibility, relative priority for finite resources, equity, and personal and societal values.

This distinction can be made clearer by considering the different levels in healthcare at which decisions are being made; by whom they are being made, and for whom they are being made.

Use of HTA at the national level

Some healthcare policy issues are resolved at national level because they require substantial infrastructure to deliver them. Population screening programmes are examples. In the UK, for instance, regular breast cancer screening by triennial mammography is offered to all women aged between 50 and 64 years. The arrangements required to do this are complex and include such elements as:

- Invitation and recall systems
- Provision of accessible mammographic facilities of a high standard
- Provision of diagnostic services for women found to have abnormalities on screening
- Treatment facilities for those in whom the diagnosis of cancer is confirmed
- Training of all health professionals providing screening
- Quality assurance.

The service requirements of such an enterprise require that population screening policy be developed nationally rather than locally. In the UK, this is the role of the National Screening Committee. Its advice to government is based upon technology assessments of each component of the programme (e.g. the screening test itself) and of the screening programme as a whole (National Screening Committee 1998).

The National Institute for Clinical Excellence (NICE) was set up in 1999 to provide authoritative national guidance to the NHS in England (Department of Health 1998). There are a number of circumstances under which the Department of Health will consider referring a technology to NICE for appraisal:

1. Is the technology (or appropriate use of the technology) likely to have a significant impact on patient care?
2. Is the technology (or appropriate use of the technology) likely to have a significant impact on other government health-related policies?
3. Is the technology (or appropriate use of the technology) likely to have a significant impact on NHS resources?
4. Is NICE likely to 'add value', e.g. by resolving uncertainty over the appropriate use of the technology?

Appraisal by NICE of health technologies is supported by technology assessment reports commissioned for the purpose by the NHS health technology assessment programme.

Examples

Some examples of technology assessment and the associated NICE guidance are indicative of the scope of the technologies considered:

- Hip replacement surgery (Fitzpatrick et al 1998, National Institute for Clinical Excellence 2000a)
- Liquid-based cytology in cervical screening (National Institute for Clinical Excellence 2000b, Payne et al 2000)
- Implantable cardioverter defibrillators (National Institute for Clinical Excellence 2001a, Parkes et al 2000)
- Orlistat and sibutramine for the management of obesity (National Institute for Clinical Excellence 2001b, 2001c; O'Meara et al 2001, 2002)
- Topotecan for ovarian cancer (Forbes et al 2001, National Institute for Clinical Excellence 2001d).

All NICE appraisals are accessible via the institute's website (www.nice.org.uk).

Use of HTA at the local level

For most health services within the NHS, service commissioning decisions are made locally. These decisions too need to be shaped by the scientific evidence of the effectiveness and cost-effectiveness of the services under consideration, but also encompass consideration of local health needs and resources. As described below, the outputs of the NHS HTA programme provide one of several HTA resources available to health service commissioners.

Use of HTA at the level of individual patient care

Although the term is not often applied to it, decision-making by an individual patient in consultation with a doctor or other health professional is also a process of appraisal. It includes the element of assessment – what treatments are available for this condition, and how effective and cost-effective are they? – but also should be influenced by issues of importance to the individual which will not be part of the scientific evidence base. Patients have individual characteristics, concurrent illnesses and preferences which must be considered when judging the applicability of that evidence. The preferred treatment option should be reached by the interplay of best evidence, professional judgement and informed individual choice. The need here is for valid and up-to-date syntheses of the evidence, accessible to the individual patient and health professional when needed. This is a challenge for information technology as well as for HTA.

Use of HTA to support decision-making in research

Knowledge of health technologies evolves over a period of time, during which the areas requiring further research will change. Even when the technology has entered clinical practice, there will be gaps in understanding which have to be filled, for example long-term effectiveness relative to alternative treatment strategies. For commissioners of research, including the HTA programme itself, it is important to have a clear view of current research needs in the field. A systematic review (or technology assessment report) will, in addition to synthesizing what is known, identify the key areas of uncertainty towards which further primary research could most usefully be directed.

As has been pointed out, screening policy must be based on a full consideration of a set of issues relating to the disease, the test, the treatment and the screening programme as a whole. The criteria favourable to an effective and appropriate screening programme have been usefully set out by the National Screening Committee (1996). For such complex policy issues, a systematic review can be particularly valuable in identifying those areas of uncertainty which are most critical to sound decision-making.

Example

This example describes findings from population screening for prostate cancer using the PSA (prostate-specific antigen) test.

PSA is produced by the prostate gland and can be measured at low concentrations in the blood of normal men. Raised levels are associated with the presence of prostate cancer, but can also be seen in non-malignant conditions such as benign prostatic hypertrophy – a very common age-related change. Marked elevation of serum PSA occurs when prostate cancer spreads outside the gland, either by local invasion or by the development of distant metastases. In principle, serum PSA might provide the basis for a screening programme to detect early prostate cancer when it is still confined to the gland and potentially curable. Systematic reviews commissioned by the HTA programme (Chamberlain et al 1997, Selley et al 1997) identified several areas of uncertainty:

- A PSA test alone cannot reliably distinguish men with early prostate cancer from men without the condition.
- Raised PSA results must be investigated further by the invasive test of prostate biopsy, and the optimum threshold value of PSA for performing such tests is uncertain.
- It is unclear what proportion of localized prostate cancers progress without treatment to cause clinical disease, or the speed at which they do so.
- The best treatment for localized prostate cancer (e.g. radical surgery, radical prostatectomy) is unknown.
- The balance of risks and benefits for a population screening programme cannot be reliably estimated in the current state of knowledge.

The main findings of these systematic reviews have since been confirmed by work commissioned by other national HTA agencies (Schersten et al 1999).

The *appraisal* of population PSA screening by the National Screening Committee (and by equivalent bodies in other countries) resulted in a policy decision not to recommend population PSA screening. In parallel, the HTA programme identified the uncertainty around the optimum treatment for localized prostate cancer as a key issue for future screening policy in this area. A large multicentre randomized control trial has now been commissioned by the HTA programme with the primary purpose of comparing three treatment strategies for screen-detected early prostate cancer: radical prostatectomy, radical radiotherapy, and active monitoring for disease progression. It will in addition yield valuable information on the natural history of the disease, the reliability of PSA testing and the acceptability of the screening and diagnostic tests to asymptomatic men (Donovan et al 2001).

HTA of diagnostic technologies

The assessment of diagnostic tests (either laboratory tests or imaging investigations) presents particular complexities. At the simplest level, the test can be studied to determine its sensitivity and specificity for the condition it is intended to identify. However, a full assessment must consider wider issues:

1. How does the performance of the test compare with the 'gold standard' for diagnosis – if there is one?

2. What impact will the use of the test have on the use of other tests? For example, what impact would the availability of CT colonography ('virtual colonoscopy') have on the use of fibreoptic colonoscopy and conventional contrast radiology of the large bowel? What would be the impact on diagnostic accuracy and the cost of investigation?

3. What would be the impact on clinical outcomes? This is essential information by which to judge the effectiveness and cost-effectiveness of the new diagnostic technology. However, 'outcome' can be defined in several ways, for example mortality, morbidity, hospital stay, quality of life. Each of these will depend not just on the diagnostic test used but on the whole sequence of diagnostic and treatment decisions made subsequently.

4. When the test uses a piece of capital equipment, its cost will be critically influenced by patterns of use of the equipment. If, for instance, a hospital has an MRI scanner in service for a range of diagnostic tests, the marginal cost of using it for a new investigation is much lower than would be the case if the full capital and revenue costs were attributable to the new test alone. In taking the key policy decisions, the use of individual diagnostic procedures may be subsidiary to the capital investment required to make them available. An example is the provision of positron emission tomography (PET), which has been the subject of an HTA scoping review (Robert and Milne 1999).

OPERATING A NATIONAL HTA PROGRAMME

After the above outline of the various functions of HTA, we can now consider the organization that is needed to run an effective HTA research programme. Three functions can be identified:

1. Defining the most important research needs
   a. Collecting potential topics for consideration
   b. Refining and prioritizing these topics
2. Commissioning the research
   a. Putting commissioning briefs out to tender
   b. Competitively selecting research proposals in the light of peer review and expert opinion

3. Ensuring delivery of successfully completed research
   a. Project monitoring and review
   b. Securing a completed research result in a form accessible to the
      end user.

This schema may be modified to meet the needs of a particular 'customer'. For example, technology assessment reports are commissioned directly from a small group of academic units which have previously been judged competent to do the work as a result of an institutional review. It would otherwise be impossible to have the work completed within the tight timescale of the NICE appraisal process. However, any commissioning process in the public sector must have adequate safeguards to ensure probity, value for money and scientific quality. Peer review is an essential component.

In the NHS programme, these various tasks are managed by the National Co-ordinating Centre for Health Technology Assessment at the University of Southampton (NCCHTA).

Defining research needs

Suggestions are gathered from many sources, such as:

- Widespread 'open channel' consultation via the HTA programme website
- Horizon scanning
- Published systematic reviews, including HTA and Cochrane reviews
- NICE appraisal reports
- Direct consultation with a wide range of affiliate organizations such as medical royal colleges and specialist groups in the health professions
- Policy sources within the Department of Health
- Reconsideration of important topics not prioritized in earlier cycles.

The 'open channel' route (www.ncchta.org) has been developed to provide the widest possible access to the prioritization process. The input screens are well supported by help screens to elicit as much information as possible about the proposed technology and why it is considered in need of assessment. Screen prompts request information on the informant's identity and area of work, and suggestions for the names of topic experts who might be consulted.

Horizon scanning is a particularly valuable source of intelligence for HTA priority-setting. It is carried out continuously by the National Horizon Scanning Centre at Birmingham University, under a contract with the NHS R&D programme. The centre's task is to identify important technologies which are thought likely to become available to the NHS over the next 1–3 years. Judgement of their likely importance is based on consideration of potential health benefit, cost impact, speed of diffusion, or other factors which may present challenges for the NHS. The NHSC provides a concise summary of the technology, completed research and research known to be in progress.

Over 1000 suggestions per year are gathered by the HTA programme from the range of sources set out above. They are collated and reduced to a shorter list of around 400 for consideration by three expert advisory panels:

- Pharmaceuticals
- Diagnostic technologies and screening
- Therapeutic procedures.

Each panel meets three times per year. The panels' membership includes a broad range of NHS and academic expertise and consumer representatives. The panels focus the proposals and, for the most promising 50 or so, request a briefing paper from NCCHTA which sets out the background to the technology, its significance to the NHS and the research which has been done or is already in progress. In the light of such information, the panel arrives at a final list of topics which go out to advertisement. By this point there will have been a decision as to whether primary or secondary research is required and a detailed commissioning brief will have been written to guide potential bidders.

The panels' role is to formulate a clear question which can be answered by research. The focus is on relatively stable technologies, i.e. those which have completed the process of technical development and are unlikely to change further during the time it takes to carry out the assessment. The question should address both effectiveness (defining outcomes important to patients) and cost-effectiveness. The comparator will be the best currently available technology used for the same indication, if there is one.

Explicit criteria are used by the Panels for setting priorities:

- What would be the benefits from an assessment, in terms of reduced uncertainty for NHS decision-makers?
- How long would it take to deliver those benefits?
- Would such an assessment represent good value for money for the NHS?
- How important is it to do an early assessment (for example, what is the current rate of diffusion of the technology into the NHS? Is there a 'window of opportunity' after which it will become very difficult either to do the research or to change practice?)
- Are there other considerations to take into account, such as government policy initiatives, disease prevalence or social/ethical issues?

Commissioning research

Invitations to submit proposals on prioritized topics are widely publicized. The media used include the scientific, medical and nursing press; the

Official Journal of the European Communities; the HTA website; R&D networks within the NHS; electronic alerts to some 1800 contacts; and direct mailshots to about 350 individuals who have registered their interest in the programme. Applicants receive the commissioning briefs, background information and detailed guidance on the application procedure. All of this material can be downloaded from the HTA website, together with an electronic proposal form.

Research groups have discretion to propose research designs which they believe will best address the question. Members of the HTA commissioning board are predominantly researchers themselves, from a range of disciplines including health services research, statistics, qualitative research and health economics. Proposals for primary research topics are usually considered first in outline. Short-listed proposals are then reconsidered as full protocols, after peer review, thereby reducing the burden on applicants at the preliminary stage.

Key considerations are the relevance of the proposal to the commissioning brief; the appropriateness of the outcome measures; the quality of the study design; the statistical power of the study, and the likelihood of achieving target recruitment. Given the scientific and clinical complexity of many topics, there may need to be some iteration between board and research group before a final protocol is recommended for funding. Every effort is made to avoid delays in reaching commissioning decisions. The board meets every 5 months – the greatest frequency which is compatible with the intervals required for peer review and other components of the process.

The working methods of the commissioning board have been progressively refined around four guiding principles:

1. Quality, both of the work commissioned and of the expert input of referees and board members
2. Openness, in the way in which decisions have been reached and communicated to applicants
3. Equity, in the treatment of all applicants
4. Efficiency, in the use of NHS resources to achieve research objectives.

Rules for the declaration of interests (personal or institutional) are explicit and enforced. Members of the board withdraw from discussion of any proposal where a conflict of interest exists.

The final step in the commissioning process is a meeting of the prioritization strategy group, chaired by the programme director and made up of the chairs of the three panels and of the commissioning board. The group's role is to reconcile the board's recommendations with the anticipated budget profile. In the event that not all can be funded, the decision is based on consideration of both the importance of the topic to the NHS and the scientific quality of the proposals. As at March 2002, 356 research projects had been commissioned at a cost of over £75 million.

The rapid commissioning route

Even with streamlined programme administration, it is not possible to respond to secondary research needs (reviews) by the standard procedures when the timescale required is of the order of months rather than the usual 1–2 years. The direct commissioning of TARs from preferred providers was initiated to fill this gap. The time interval between topic identification and report delivery is about 6 months. There is contracted capacity for approximately 50 TARs per year in a network of seven academic centres throughout the UK. Most of the topics handled by this route, but not all, are new technologies which have been referred by the Department of Health to NICE for appraisal.

Ensuring delivery of successfully completed research

At any time there will be over 100 HTA projects in progress. They range from complex multicentre trials lasting up to 10 years to systematic reviews where completion is essential within 6 months. The task of monitoring is to facilitate the successful delivery of high-quality research, on time and within budget.

All research funding is to some extent speculative investment. The risks are broadly of two kinds. The first is a failure of process: missed milestones, under-recruitment, or poor data quality, for example. Such failures are in principle avoidable by sound planning, a well thought out protocol and good project management. The second risk is that the successfully completed project yields no new knowledge that can be used to improve healthcare. This is an inescapable hazard of all research; if the outcome were known in advance, there would be no reason to do the study. However, it is rare for HTA research to yield no worthwhile knowledge. Clear evidence that a technology is not more effective or cost-effective than existing interventions (or none) should prevent its diffusion or lead to its discontinuation with the release of resources for other things. Less commonly, the question may have been superseded, or fully answered elsewhere, during the course of the work. Thorough horizon scanning and liaison with other funders should make this unlikely.

Project monitoring is concerned with minimizing the first type of risk. Its role is not to further burden the researchers with bureaucracy but to provide support, encouragement and the benefit of experience gained elsewhere in the programme.

It is usually possible to make some prior estimation of the investment risk associated with an individual project and to tailor the intensity of monitoring appropriately. Some research projects are intrinsically more difficult to deliver than others – for instance if they depend on the collaboration of many participants to achieve target recruitment. Protracted or expensive projects can likewise be seen as at higher than average risk of failure. A recurring theme in all primary research (particularly of the complex and multifaceted kind common in HTA) is failure to recruit sufficient patients. The reasons for this are usually multiple. Quite commonly, there is incomplete advance knowledge of the number of patients who will fall within the study inclusion criteria. The willingness of clinicians to randomize patients is to some extent affected by service pressures. The willingness of patients to agree to participate can be hard to estimate in advance and is likely to depend in part on what will be demanded of recruits. Delays in obtaining ethical approval, the agreement of host institutions or in the recruitment of key support staff can all adversely affect recruitment rate.

Progress reports at regular intervals will give information on actual as against planned recruitment rates (best represented as cumulative graphs). It is important to identify recruitment shortfall as early as possible, to establish the factors contributing to it and to take corrective action quickly. This might include the inclusion of additional centres of recruitment, or movement of resources from under-performing to more successful centres. A recruitment rate below target should generally be anticipated, with an agreed contingency plan ready to be activated immediately. That provides the best prospect of reaching target sample size within the agreed study duration and budget.

For demanding projects, where there is a real possibility that the design may not be feasible to implement on the required scale, a pilot phase may be commissioned. The funding of the main study will then be conditional on evidence of feasibility.

Example

This example concerns the feasibility of identifying and randomizing adequate numbers of men with localized prostate cancer to a trial comparing active monitoring, radical prostatectomy and radical radiotherapy.

The rationale for such a study has been described above. Areas of uncertainty in planning the research include:

- The proportion of healthy men willing to accept an invitation for a PSA screening test
- The detection rate for gland-localized prostate cancer in this population
- The proportion of men so diagnosed who will accept randomization to any of three very different management strategies
- The proportion of men who will accept the treatment randomly allocated, having consented to be randomized.

Successful completion of a 2-year feasibility phase yielded accurate data on each of these uncertainties. It also allowed the communication and uptake of information in the trial setting to be carefully analysed by qualitative techniques, so that trial methods could be refined. The main trial was then initiated with considerably greater confidence in its feasibility (Donovan et al 2001).

Risk-stratification of projects is also used to select studies in progress for site visits. The opportunity to examine the progress of the work in detail with the researchers is invaluable, and allows possible protocol modifications to be discussed if necessary. Because of the nature of primary HTA research, embedded as it is within service delivery, there is much to be gained from a good working partnership between the funding body and the investigators.

The draft final report of each project is submitted for editorial review with the aim of publication in the monograph series *Health Technology Assessment*. It will be reviewed by at least three independent experts, by panel and board members familiar with the prioritization of the topic and the commissioning of the protocol, and often a relevant consumer organization. Editors review the manuscript and reviewers' comments, provide feedback to authors and request a revised draft where necessary.

The series is indexed in the international bibliographic databases (MEDLINE, EMBASE). In addition to the hard copy version, the full text is available both on the Internet (www.ncchta.org) and as a cumulative CD-ROM issued bi-annually. As shown in Figure 3.1, electronic access is a major route of dissemination. Approximately half of the demand is from outside the UK (Fig. 3.2).

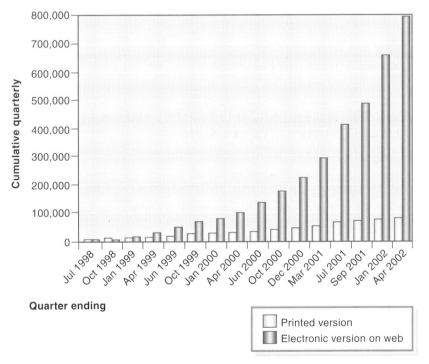

Figure 3.1 Distribution of HTA monographs as hard copy and as electronic page downloads via the Internet, by quarter, 1998–2002.

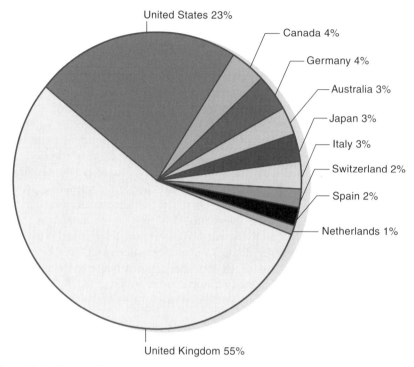

United States 23%

Canada 4%

Germany 4%

Australia 3%

Japan 3%

Italy 3%

Switzerland 2%

Spain 2%

Netherlands 1%

United Kingdom 55%

Figure 3.2 Source of download requests for a monograph (Hoare et al 2000) on the NCCHTA website (top 10 countries, $n = 2849$).

MAKING HTA RESEARCH OUTPUTS AVAILABLE TO DECISION-MAKERS IN THE NHS

The process described above was designed to deliver high-quality research findings, relevant to the needs of the NHS, into the public domain. One additional task for a national HTA programme is to ensure as far as is possible that the research outputs are brought to the attention of those decision-makers who are able to implement them. Implementation is not an R&D function but is of course essential if research investment is to yield value. Ideally, key end users will have been party to the commissioning process and will have given thought to the practical implications of the results.

The working relationship between HTA and a defined end user has been productively explored since the setting up of the National Institute for Clinical Excellence in April 1999. The role of NICE is, among other things, to be the source of guidance to the NHS on the appropriate use of individual technologies through its appraisal committee. In many ways the functional links between the HTA programme and NICE serve as a paradigm for the inter-relationship of assessment and appraisal in healthcare. Assessment gathers the available evidence on effectiveness and cost-effectiveness in a rigorous and unbiased way, using transparent research methodology. Appraisal translates that knowledge into practical application by a judgement which is legitimately informed by other considerations such as feasibility, equity and relative priority within the specific context of the NHS. To meet the requirements of NICE, the HTA programme has developed a new format of research output – the TAR – and the rapid mode of commissioning as previously described.

There is, however, a far wider constituency of customers for HTA. Only a small proportion of decisions in healthcare can – or should – be the subject of national guidance. At regional and local level, a multitude of questions concerning the provision and commissioning of health services must be made. In the consultation between individual patients and their clinical advisers, there is a need to know the existing evidence for the effectiveness and relative cost-effectiveness of alternative means of diagnosis and treatment. There are some 250 million consultations annually in primary care in the NHS, for example. How is HTA to be made accessible on this scale?

The challenge has two elements. The first is to achieve adequate and up-to-date coverage of the range of interventions used in modern healthcare. The second is concerned with knowledge management – getting information to where it is needed, when it is needed, in an organization which is unique in its scale and in the complexity of its role. The latter generic issue will not be considered further here.

As regards the former challenge, it is unrealistic to hope that a single national programme will be able to provide complete and contemporaneous topic coverage across the whole broad scope of HTA. This is the reason why such effort is put into the prioritization of topics to be commissioned. However, the enquirer whose specific need is not covered by the existing portfolio of the NHS HTA programme can access a range of alternative national and international resources through the Internet. These include:

- The Cochrane Database of Systematic Reviews
- The Database of Abstracts of Reviews of Effectiveness (DARE)
- The NHS Economic Evaluation Database (NEED)
- The international database of HTA reports held by INAHTA (the International Network of Agencies for HTA).

Each of the first three is funded wholly or in part by the NHS R&D programme. The website of the NHS Centre for Reviews and Dissemination at the University of York is a valuable gateway to all these resources which collectively provide several thousand reviews of high quality (http://www.york.ac.uk/inst/crd/).

Such a multiplicity of reviews greatly increases topic coverage, but also provides a degree of replication which is a valuable safeguard. One of the characteristics of unbiased research is that it should be reproducible by independent groups using the available evidence at a point in time. This is particularly important when large national policy initiatives are being decided. Two examples from the field of population screening illustrate the point. For PSA testing to detect early prostate cancer in the general population, independent HTA reviews carried out in seven countries concluded that there was no adequate evidence that such screening would be effective in reducing mortality and morbidity (Schersten et al 1999). For breast cancer mammographic screening, by contrast, independent reviews of the evidence have not been entirely consistent. The main point of contention has been around the quality assessment of the various screening trials which between them constitute the international evidence base on the topic. These inconsistencies have been thoroughly explored in scientific debate (Gotzsche & Olsen 2000, Health Council of the Netherlands 2002). Ultimately, a policy decision for or against population screening by mammography is a matter for appraisal. Technology assessment can inform that judgement but not directly determine the decision. As Churchill put it succinctly, in another context: 'Scientists should be on tap, not on top.'

SUMMARY AND CONCLUSION

This chapter has given an overview of the NHS HTA research programme. In so doing it has focused upon the development and implementation of the programme. The research cycle (see Ch. 1) has been considered from developing ideas based upon healthcare needs through to managing the research activity and disseminating findings. In providing much needed evidence for healthcare delivery this programme illustrates the success of the NHS R&D strategy in that the ideas for the research are developed from identifiable health needs in a well-coordinated way. This programme, alongside the other national programmes referred to above can be seen as the realization of the NHS R&D vision for research outlined in Chapter 2. The continuing evolution of activity has demonstrated it is possible to focus research developments upon healthcare needs.

REFERENCES

Bricker L, Garcia J, Henderson J et al 2000 Ultrasound screening in pregnancy: a systematic review of the clinical effectiveness, cost-effectiveness and women's views. Health Technology Assessment 4(16): i–vi, 1–193
Brocklebank D, Ram F, Wright J et al 2001 Comparison of the effectiveness of inhaler devices in asthma and chronic obstructive airways disease: a systematic review of the literature. Health Technology Assessessment 5(26): 1–149
Bruce J, Russell E M, Mollison J, Krukowski Z H 2001 The measurement and monitoring of surgical adverse events. Health Technology Assessment 5(22): 1–186
Chamberlain J, Melia J, Moss S, Brown J 1997 The diagnosis, management, treatment and costs of prostate cancer in England and Wales. Health Technology Assessment 1(3): 1–194

Cuzick J, Sasieni P, Davies P et al 1999 A systematic review of the role of human papilloma virus testing within a cervical screening programme. Health Technology Assessment 3(14): i–iv, 1–196

Delaney B, Moayyedi P, Deeks J et al 2000 The management of dyspepsia: a systematic review. Health Technology Assessment 4(39): iii–v, 1–189

Department of Health 1998 A first class service: quality in the new NHS. Department of Health, London

Department of Health 2002 Health technology assessment programme annual report, 2002. Department of Health, London

Donovan J, Frankel S, Neal D, Hamdy F 2001 Screening for prostate cancer in the UK: seems to be creeping in by the back door. British Medical Journal 323: 763–764

Fairbank L, O'Meara S, Renfrew M, Woolridge M, Sowden A, Lister-Sharp D 2000 A systematic review to evaluate the effectiveness of interventions to promote the initiation of breastfeeding. Health Technology Assessment 4(25): 1–171

Fitzpatrick R, Shortall E, Sculpher M et al 1998 Primary total hip replacement surgery: a systematic review of outcomes and modelling of cost-effectiveness associated with different prostheses. Health Technology Assessment 2(20): 1–64

Forbes C, Shirran L, Bagnall A-M, Duffy S, ter Riet G 2001 A rapid and systematic review of the clinical effectiveness and cost-effectiveness of topotecan for ovarian cancer. Health Technology Assessment 5(28): 1–110

Gotzsche P, Olsen O 2000 Is screening for breast cancer with mammography justifiable? Lancet 355: 129–134

Health Council of the Netherlands 2002 The benefit of population screening for breast cancer with mammography. Health Council of the Netherlands, The Hague

Hoare C, Li Wan Po A, Williams H 2000 Systematic review of treatments for atopic eczema. Health Technology Assessment 4(37): 1–191

National Institute for Clinical Excellence 2000a Guidance on the selection of prostheses for primary total hip replacement. National Institute for Clinical Excellence, Appraisal Guidance (http://www.nice.org.uk)

National Institute for Clinical Excellence 2000b Guidance on the use of liquid based cytology for cervical screening. National Institute for Clinical Excellence, Appraisal Guidance (http://www.nice.org.uk)

National Institute for Clinical Excellence 2001a Guidance on the use of implantable cardioverter defibrillators for arrhythmias. National Institute for Clinical Excellence, Appraisal Guidance (http://www.nice.org.uk)

National Institute for Clinical Excellence 2001b Guidance on the use of orlistat for the treatment of obesity in adults. National Institute for Clinical Excellence, Appraisal Guidance (http://www.nice.org.uk)

National Institute for Clinical Excellence 2001c Guidance on the use of sibutramine for the treatment of obesity in adults. National Institute for Clinical Excellence, Appraisal Guidance (http://www.nice.org.uk)

National Institute for Clinical Excellence 2001d Guidance on the use of topotecan for the treatment of advanced ovarian cancer. National Institute for Clinical Excellence, Appraisal Guidance (http://www.nice.org.uk)

National Screening Committee 1996 The National Screening Committee's criteria for appraising the viability, effectiveness and appropriateness of a screening programme. Department of Health, London

National Screening Committee 1998 First report of the National Screening Committee. Department of Health, London

O'Meara S, Riemsma R, Shirran L, Mather L, ter Riet G 2001 A rapid and systematic review of the clinical effectiveness and cost-effectiveness of orlistat in the management of obesity. Health Technology Assessment 5(18): 1–81

O'Meara S, Riemsma R, Shirran L, Mather L, ter Riet G 2002 The clinical effectiveness and cost-effectiveness of sibutramine in the management of obesity: a technology assessment. Health Technology Assessment 6(6): 1–97

Parkes J, Bryant J, Milne R 2000 Implantable cardioverter defibrillators: arrhythmias. A rapid and systematic review. Health Technology Assessment 4(26): 1–69

Payne N, Chilcott J, McGoogan E 2000 Liquid-based cytology in cervical screening: a rapid and systematic review. Health Technology Assessment 4(18): 1–73

Pembrey M, Barnicoat A, Carmichael B, Bobrow M, Turner G 2001 An assessment of screening strategies for fragile X syndrome in the UK. Health Technology Assessment 5(7): 1–95

Robert G, Milne R 1999 Positron emission tomography: establishing priorities for health technology assessment. Health Technology Assessment 3(16): 1–54

Schersten T, Baile M, Asua J, Jonsson E 1999 Prostate cancer screening: evidence synthesis and update, statement of findings. International Network of Agencies for Health Technology Assessment, Stockholm

Selley S, Donovan J, Faulkner A, Coast J, Gillatt D 1997 Diagnosis, management and screening of early localised prostate cancer. Health Technology Assessment 1(2): i, 1–96

Spiegelhalter D, Myles J, Jones D R, Abrams K R 2000 Bayesian methods in health technology assessment: a review. Health Technology Assessment 4(38): 1–130

Sutton A, Abrams K, Jones D, Sheldon T, Song F 1998 Systematic reviews of trials and other studies. Health Technology Assessment 2(19): 1–276

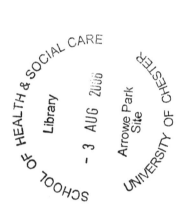

4

Managing the local agenda: planning to get research/evidence-based care into practice

Maggie Griffiths   Jenny Clark

Editors' comment

This chapter examines the concept of evidence-based practice from the perspective of an NHS trust. It reviews the political context within which NHS trusts currently operate and identifies the factors that have influenced the drive towards clinical effectiveness in healthcare delivery. The notion of clinical governance is explored in depth and readers are offered a wealth of information relating to how and where they can access the relevant evidence whereby to examine their own practice. The chapter stresses that practitioners need to be not only informed of best practice in given situations but also empowered to make changes to their practice in the light of the evidence. To that end the chapter examines the concept of change management and offers readers a range of helpful practices based on relevant change theory that would assist clinicians to implement changes in practice.

INTRODUCTION

The NHS Executive (1996) summarized the three main functions in achieving clinical effectiveness in practice under the following headings:

- Inform
- Change
- Monitor

Firstly, it is essential to ensure that all clinicians, patients and managers are aware of the importance of clinical effectiveness and have access to the best available evidence upon which to base their care. Secondly, they need to be facilitated to use this information to review their practice and to make changes as necessary. Finally, they need to monitor the effects of the changes to ensure that they result in real improvements in the quality of healthcare. This chapter will address two of the above aspects by examining some of the current influences on NHS organisations and discussing some practical steps that can help in introducing research findings to change practice and improve patient care.

CURRENT INFLUENCES ON NHS ORGANIZATIONS

To set the scene, the first part of the chapter will look briefly at the policy changes following the election of the Labour government in 1997. It will then examine in more detail the concept of clinical governance and its impact on organizations.

During the early 1990s, the NHS suffered a loss of public confidence. This was due to various factors including an increasing number of people waiting for treatment, variation in services across the country, rising numbers of complaints and a number of high-profile investigations into failures of the service, most notably the Bristol inquiry chaired by Sir Ian Kennedy. This was set up to inquire into the management of the care of children receiving complex cardiac surgical services at the Bristol Royal Infirmary (BRI) between 1984 and 1995 and relevant related issues. Its remit was also to form conclusions from these events and to make recommendations that could help to secure high-quality care across the NHS (Bristol Royal Infirmary 2001). It is important to note that the final summary of the report states that:

It is an account of people who cared greatly about human suffering, and were dedicated and well-motivated. Sadly, some lacked insight and their behaviour was flawed. Many failed to communicate with each other, and to work together effectively for the interests of their patients. There was a lack of leadership and teamwork … [this combination of circumstances] owed as much to general failings of the NHS at the time than to any individual failing. (p. 1)

In the general election campaign of 1997, the NHS was a major area of discussion for the main political parties. Following the election of the Labour Party, the White Paper *The New NHS: Modern and Dependable* (Department of Health 1997) was published. The Consultation Paper *A First Class Service: Quality in the NHS* (Department of Health 1998) was published the following year. The documents outlined a 10-year modernization plan for the NHS. The main message of this plan was that patients are at the centre of the service and should receive high-quality care delivered by appropriately trained staff using evidence-based practice. The White Paper noted that:

There is concern when it is thought patients are being denied potentially beneficial new treatments. But a wider, if less reported, concern is the number of patients being denied proved treatments because of a delay by health professionals and managers in acting on published evidence. The time lag between research paper and bedside practice means many patients are being denied effective therapy. (Department of Health 1997, p. 6)

A First Class Service (Department of Health 1998) set out in more detail the framework for quality improvement in the NHS. The main elements of the framework included:

• The publication of clear national standards for services and treatments through national service frameworks

- The establishment of a National Institute for Clinical Excellence (NICE)
- Local delivery of high-quality healthcare through clinical governance
- Modernized professional self-regulation and a commitment to lifelong learning for healthcare professionals
- The monitoring of the NHS by the Commission for Health Improvement (CHI)
- A framework for assessing performance
- A national survey of patients and users to monitor their experiences.

The *NHS Plan* (Department of Health 2000a) identified how these reforms would be achieved. The plan's main areas included changing the way the beds in the acute sector were used, plus an increase in intermediate and respite beds and the development of ambulatory care services; new roles and responsibilities for healthcare professionals and changing ways of working; IT to support the changes and provide effective and timely information for staff; an increase in resources year on year; and the development of a number of national service frameworks. The frameworks outline standards of care for people with a range of conditions, including cancer and heart disease, that inform patients, clients and carers about the way services are to be delivered.

The Health Act 1999 (Department of Health 1999) paved the way for the establishment of NICE, CHI and a system of clinical governance underpinned by modernized professional self-regulation and lifelong learning. It also included, for the first time, a statutory duty for quality for healthcare organizations and the people that lead them. This meant that both clinicians and managers are responsible for the quality of healthcare provided.

NICE and CHI were set up and started to operate fully from April 1999. They cover the NHS in England and Wales. More information on the NHS in Wales is available on its website, http://www.wales.nhs.uk.

The role of NICE is to give patients, healthcare professionals and the public advice on current 'best practice' in healthcare, based on reliable evidence. Further information on its work, and the guidelines it has produced so far can be found on its website, http://www.nice.org.uk. CHI is a non-departmental public body whose aim according to its website is:

to improve the quality of healthcare within the NHS. CHI will raise standards by:

- Assessing every NHS organisation and making its findings public
- Investigating where there is serious failure
- Checking that the NHS is following national guidelines
- Advising the NHS on best practice.

More information on its working and the monitoring reports it produces on the organizations it has visited can be found on its website, http://www.chi.nhs.uk. It will have an expanded role from April 2004 and be known as the Commission for Healthcare Audit and Inspection (CHAI).

Scotland has different arrangements for the roles of NICE and CHI. Further information on the arrangements in Scotland is available on http://www.nhshealthquality.org. Northern Ireland is not currently covered by these arrangements although closer working relationships may develop as part of devolution arrangements for the province. More information on the NHS in Northern Ireland is available on www.n-i.nhs.uk.

In 2000 a Consultation Paper, *Shifting the Balance of Power* (Department of Health 2000b), was published which outlined a further restructuring of the NHS with the abolition of the NHS Executive regional offices and the establishment of strategic health authorities. There were also increased powers for primary care trusts and the abolition of community health councils. These changes resulted in the NHS Reform and Health Care Professionals Act (HMSO 2002). This legislation also included changes in healthcare professional's registration and re-registration, which will have an effect on both an organization and an individual's responsibility for professional development.

CLINICAL GOVERNANCE

What is clinical governance? In *A First Class Service* (Department of Health 1998) clinical governance was described as: 'A framework through which NHS organisations are accountable for continuously improving the quality of their services and safeguarding high standards of care by creating an environment in which excellence in clinical care will flourish' (Department of Health 1998, p. 33). Holt (1999) notes that the clinical governance framework merges responsibility for clinical and managerial leadership.

Walshe et al (2000) offer still further understanding and describe clinical governance as being:

At the centre of the NHS quality reforms. It involves establishing clear lines of responsibility and accountability for quality in NHS organisations, putting a comprehensive programme of quality improvement activity in place, and having robust arrangements for identifying and remedying risks and poor performance. It is generally accepted that clinical governance demands a shift in the values, culture and leadership of the NHS, to place greater focus on the quality of clinical care and to make it easier to bring about improvement and changes in clinical practice. (Walshe et al 2000, p. 1)

Dale et al (1998) identified four major pillars of clinical governance. They are:

- Improving clinical effectiveness
- Professional development
- Continuous quality improvement
- Risk management.

So how do these changes affect practitioners at a local level? Does the introduction of clinical governance help clinicians deliver high-quality care to patients and clients? On one hand the introduction of these reforms should help in improving clinical effectiveness and making changes to practice, if required, easier to achieve. They can act as a catalyst for change. Extra resources have been put into the NHS and quality of care has become part of the manager's as well as the clinician's agenda. New facilities are being built and leadership and teamwork are being promoted as part of the NHS Leadership Centre with the Modernisation Agency. But the reality may be very different from the rhetoric. As Bate (1994) notes: 'Change is a highly complex business, difficult to understand and because of its non-linear nature almost impossible to deal with systematically or to write about convincingly' (p. 3). Or, put another way, first there was the plan; then there is the operational strategy and the implementation, which is the difficult part. As General Norman Schwarzkopf once remarked, 'The truth of the matter is that you always know the right thing to do. The hard part is doing it' (Bate 2001).

THE EFFECTIVENESS OF CLINICAL GOVERNANCE

There have been a number of studies that have examined the implementation of clinical governance. They include Firth-Cozens (1999) who reported that 69% of the sample asked (220 healthcare professionals representing primary and secondary care) had heard of the term clinical governance but detailed knowledge was rare. Preston & Baker (2000) sent out a postal questionnaire to 506 local groups in England and Wales and of the 329 (65%) that responded 316 (96%) had or were developing a clinical governance strategy. The main problems that were reported were lack of resources and time.

The Royal College of Nursing (RCN) undertook a series of discussion groups in 1998, 1999 and 2000. The third round took place with clinical nurses, senior managers and clinical governance facilitators (Currie & Loftus-Hills 2002). Three key issues emerged in all three rounds of the groups. They were:

- The need to raise awareness of clinical governance at local level to staff working on wards and departments.
- The need to address and change the culture of the organizations to make them more receptive to the clinical governance framework, thus enabling staff to work in an environment that does not blame but rather learns from incidents and complaints.
- The need for greater partnerships between patients and professionals, clinicians and managers.

These findings broadly agree with Walshe et al (2000) who examined the implementation of clinical governance within 47 trusts in the West Midlands. The research, conducted between April 1999 and May 2000, reported that there had been some short-term progress in the implementation of clinical governance with the positive signs being that trusts were changing but that more work was needed. The report also noted that there was little evidence that clinicians had more than, at best, an awareness of clinical governance but more resources and attention were needed at ward and departmental level to make clinical governance happen. They also found little evidence of explicit actions designed to bring that cultural change about or even to begin a cultural transition. NHS trusts are very complex organizations which do not have a single organizational culture and clinical governance seems to require a major cultural change, which is always difficult to achieve. Their findings seem to show that there is some awareness of the concepts but the implementation is still far from mainstream.

ACCESSING THE EVIDENCE

Information for clinicians regarding best practice is available in different formats and accessed in a variety of settings. Where to look depends on the type of question that needs to be answered. It is important to note that: 'Evidence based practice is not simply a pragmatic, logical process, involving access to, and the subsequent use of, best research evidence. There is an interplay of multiple factors that influence decisions about patient care; an amalgamation of evidence, context, expert practice/experience and patient preferences and wishes' (Closs & Cheater 1999, p. 17). There are helpful guides to help find up-to-date information on best practice, as McKenna et al (1999) argue: 'The possibility that a person requiring health care in the latter part of the twentieth century can receive a service that is not based on best practice is unacceptable to most people' (McKenna et al 1999, p. 39).

For the majority of nurses and allied health professionals information can be obtained from books, journals, on-line databases and the Internet. Each have their advantages and disadvantages. Books can take up to 2 years to be published and so it is not guaranteed that developments that occur in the publishing period will be included. The number of journals available to healthcare professionals has grown enormously in recent years and may be available on-line. Some of the evidence-based journals (e.g. *Evidence-Based Nursing, Evidence-Based Mental Health, Evidence-Based Medicine*) provide useful guides on how to access information on best practice.

On-line bibliographic databases include: the Cumulated Index to Nursing and Allied Health Literature (CINAHL), which is a general database from the USA (http://www.cinahl.com/); Medline, a large general purpose database also from America (http://www.medline.com), and Embase, a general database from the Excerpta Medica in the Netherlands (http://www.embase.com). Information on how to search these databases is available in a series of articles from *Evidence-Based Nursing* (DiCenso et al 1998) or by contacting your local NHS librarian.

The Internet has revolutionized the availability of information for health-care professionals as it provides a huge source of information readily available to both healthcare professionals and patients. The quality of the information, however, may vary. Considerable care is needed in order to get the most appropriate information that is available; check the source, talk to a colleague and apply some of the principles that you would apply to any other information sources.

From a research perspective, valuable sources available include the Cochrane Collaboration. The Cochrane Collaboration is an international net-work of healthcare professionals plus lay people who produce and maintain systematic reviews of the effects of interventions in healthcare. Further infor-mation is available on http://www.cochrane.co.uk and http://www.jr2.ox. ac.uk/bandolier.

These developments over recent years mean that access to communica-tion for the healthcare professional is vastly superior to what existed before. While it must be acknowledged that organizations such as Cochrane and the Bandolier have always provided good published output, dissemination of this in written form meant it took a relatively long time to filter down the healthcare hierarchy. Information availability on the NHS Intranet means that information is available to all healthcare professionals at the same time.

The National Research Register

This is a register of ongoing and recently completed research funded by, or of interest to, staff of the NHS and as such provides a useful source of infor-mation both for those wishing to find out about research that has been done in their context as well as ongoing work that may help inform local devel-opments. Further information is available via the Department of Health website, www.doh.gov.uk.

The National Electronic Library for Health

This is available via the Internet. It is currently working with NHS libraries to develop a digital library for NHS staff, patients and the public. More information is available from their website, www.nelh.nhs.uk.

It is important to remember when getting information (e.g. photocopying articles or obtaining information from the Internet) that issues of storage and retrieval also need to be considered, as effective retrieval is linked to effective practice. Various systems can be used to help organize resources ranging from card indexes to software packages, depending on individual preferences, and advice can be obtained from librarians or research depart-ments in trusts or universities.

The issue of how nurses in acute care settings access information has been examined recently by Thompson et al (2001) whose study examined the accessibility of research-based knowledge for nurses in the UK. They found that nurses' experiences in a clinical speciality were positively associated with a perception that human sources, such as clinical nurse specialists, link nurses, doctors and experienced clinical colleagues, are more accessible than text-based sources. This is an interesting finding considering the amount of investment that has been made in information technology in recent years within the NHS and the different developments aimed at ensuring improved access for research findings. Thompson and colleagues argue, however, that: 'Providing critical appraisal skills, developing nurses' research implementation skills and forging complex strategies of research utilisation will ultimately prove fruitless if not based on an understanding of how real nurses (as opposed to academics' visions of nurses) access information for real clinical problems in real-time' (Thompson et al 2001, p. 12).

There is a plethora of guidelines, frameworks and databases to check, and sometimes it is not the information that is lacking for the busy practitioner but the time to read and reflect on the information gathered and its impact on practice.

INTRODUCING RESEARCH FINDINGS TO CHANGE PRACTICE AND IMPROVE PATIENT CARE

We have looked at the obstacles in this area but what is the evidence about how to overcome them? What works and what does not in the real world of competing priorities, resource limitations and changing consumer demands? Evidence is emerging on ways of implementing evidence-based care and this has been summarized in an effectiveness bulletin from York University (1999) outlining successful strategies for change. It provides an overview of various strategies and approaches to changing professional practice, and aims to provide useful advice to people who are involved in this area. More information can be found on their website, www.york.ac.uk/inst/crd.

In a recent evaluation report from Dunning et al (1999) for the King's Fund the issues of change in clinical settings were explored in 16 Promoting Action on Clinical Effectiveness (PACE) studies across England. The projects were set up in 1995 and completed in 1998. The findings conclude that change can be achieved if sound evidence is available and a project approach to manage the implementation is planned. The findings report that change is not, as has already been noted, a linear task, 'but rather a group of complex, inter-related tasks which require skill and dexterity to manage a satisfactory conclusion' (Dunning et al 1999, p. 8). Their findings support other research, which reported that a multifaceted approach is required (Rogers 1994).

Harvey et al (2002) reported:

That implementation is explained as a function of the relation between evidence (research evidence, clinical experience and patient preferences), context (culture, leadership and measurement) and facilitation (characteristics, role and style).

The three elements of evidence, context and facilitation are each positioned on a low to high continuum. We suggest that the most successful implementation occurs when evidence is scientifically robust (high) and when there is appropriate facilitation of change using the skills of external and internal facilitators. (Harvey et al 2002, p. 2)

In summary, there are different approaches to the implementation of best practice. It is dependant on the type of changes that are being considered, good communication between the team members and relevant preparation and planning of both finding the evidence and a strategy of how to introduce it. This strategy should also include a plan of what to do when people disagree or refuse to accept the evidence. These steps do not guarantee success but have been found to be effective in the primary and secondary sectors. Everyone agrees there are no easy answers in this type of work but a good team and a sense of humour are among the best tools for the job!

THE MANAGEMENT OF CHANGE

Life does not exist in a vacuum and every day of our lives we are exposed to change and to the influence of others who seek to change the way we think and behave, explicitly, implicitly, overtly or covertly. Change is all around us and as we are required to live with change it is to our benefit that we learn how to manage it effectively. This is just as important for the small but essential changes occurring in our everyday practice as it is for the larger strategic organizational changes.

The theoretical foundations of change theory are somewhat complex, as traditionally change management has drawn on a wide range of social science disciplines to inform its practice. Burns (1996), however, does try to categorize the main perspectives upon which change management theory currently stands. He suggests three predominant perspectives or schools of thought, each one identifying the major focus of attention in the change process, namely the individual, the group and the system.

The individual perspective

This perspective, as the name implies, concentrates on the part played by individuals in the change process. Behaviourist theory stipulates that all behaviour is learned and that the individual is a passive recipient of external stimuli. Through a process of conditioning first demonstrated by Pavlov (1927) individuals can be taught to respond to stimuli. Positive rewards promote repetition of the behaviour while behaviours that go unrewarded or ignored are dropped. The work of Pavlov was the foundation upon which current behaviour modification practices have been developed where change in behaviour can be manipulated by reinforcing stimuli. There are many that would criticize this approach as it suggests that human beings are like automated robots that respond solely to external stimuli. However, an important message does emerge from this theory that is worthy of consideration when attempting to bring change about in clinical practice, and that is to remember that individuals will respond well to positive reinforcement. An atmosphere of encouragement and positive feedback created by the change agent is much more likely to foster long-term internalization of the change into normal practice than when no such feedback is given.

Gestalt theorists view the role played by individuals in the change process differently from the behaviourist. They suggest that behaviour is not just the result of external stimuli to which a person is subjected but rather the way in which individuals use reason to interpret the stimuli to which they are subjected. They advocate that individuals can be encouraged to change behaviour by increasing their understanding of both themselves and the change situation. Again there are important lessons here for the would-be change agent seeking to change practice in the light of appropriate evidence. The creation of a culture that fosters debate and seeks to discuss openly relevant research findings in clinical practice is more likely to experience staff who have a greater willingness to change due to their increased awareness of all the issues involved.

The group perspective

Groups are often more powerful in change situations than individuals. Those theorists (Lewin 1958, French & Bell 1984) who advocate the group approach to change would argue that within organizations individuals do not work in isolation but rather are members of teams or work groups and are therefore constantly subjected to the collective norms and values of the group. They would suggest that these group norms and values take precedence over individual norms and values due to the fact that individuals are exposed to group pressures to conform with the group and these are very powerful stimuli. Theorists supporting the group dynamics approach to change would therefore argue that it is of little benefit trying to change individual behaviour as the individual will always be over-ridden by group pressures to conform. This theory has been very influential in modern day organizational development (OD) strategy where greater emphasis has been placed on teams and expert groups to move the organization forward rather than individuals. Change agents need to be aware of the powerful influence of the team in the facilitation of change and seek to influence key members of the team who will then drive change forward.

The systems perspective

Systems theorists advocate a macro approach to change and suggest that the main focus of attention should be the organization in its entirety and not the individual or the groups within it. Systems theorists Burns & Stalker (1961) and Lawrence & Lorsch (1967) among others suggest that all organizations are open systems that are made up of many sub-systems. The sub-systems interact with one another and failure in one sub-system will affect another sub-system bringing about disequilibrium in the organization. The important factor is therefore to ensure that synergy exists between the sub-systems. Systems theory contributes to our understanding of successful change strategy by emphasizing the need to take a holistic view of the whole organization rather than just concentrating on the individuals or groups within it. The systems theory approach would take into consideration the fact that changes in the practices in one part of the organization without considering the impact of the change on the other parts of the whole organization could be detrimental overall. An important message here is that no change should be viewed in isolation and the knock-on effects of the change to other departments within the organization should always be considered prior to implementation. This assumes even greater importance in organizations that support matrix style structures and where the emphasis is on expert teams and the devolution of decision-making and resources away from top management down to the workforce. This can predispose towards a degree of introversion in decision-making and a failure to recognize the impact of local change on the wider organization as a whole.

The three perspectives described above should not be viewed in isolation from one another but rather as complementary to one another in the advice that they offer to change agents seeking to bring about change in practice. An important consideration could be to determine the nature of the change to be implemented and at what level within the organization it rests. Does the change primarily affect the individual, groups or the organization as a whole? This should guide your choice of the most appropriate approach to take. However, a note of caution is that it is almost impossible to separate these three into disparate groups and therefore the contingency approach incorporating elements of all three approaches is probably the most beneficial overall.

LEVELS OF CHANGE: PARTICIPATIVE VERSUS DIRECTIVE CHANGE

It could be useful at this point to increase our understanding of the levels of change and change cycles. Hersey & Blanchard (1988) identify four levels of change, namely:

- Knowledge
- Attitudes
- Individual behaviour
- Group behaviour.

Knowledge is traditionally the easiest aspect to change as it can be influenced by reading a book or listening to an inspired speaker. Attitudes involve our emotions and deeply held beliefs and are therefore more difficult to change than knowledge. Changing individual behaviour comes next in the level of difficulty. Individuals may know the facts and embrace fully the reasons for a specific change but still not change their behaviour for a variety of reasons. A perceived lack of skill to perform confidently certain tasks associated with the proposed change could be an influencing factor. Finally, changing group behaviour is the most difficult to achieve due to the sheer numbers involved. Hersey & Blanchard (1988) also identify two change cycles from the four levels of change, which they entitle:

- Participative change
- Directive change.

Participative change (Fig. 4.1)

The participative change cycle starts with providing knowledge which in turn influences a change in attitudes that influences an individual to change his or her behaviour. The individual then acts as a change agent and sells the change to colleagues who in turn are influenced to change their behaviour. This is a bottom-up approach to change which tends to be rather slow

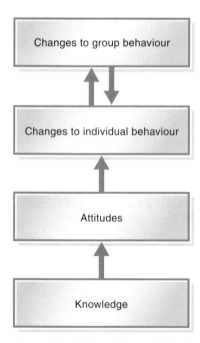

Figure 4.1   Participatory change (adapted from Hersey & Blanchard 1988).

and evolutionary; however, the change does tend to be owned by the work-force once it is implemented and has a greater chance of internalization into working practices long term. This change cycle invariably requires a flat-tened matrix style organizational structure with an emphasis on task or expert power to operate successfully.

Directive change

Directive change occurs in the opposite direction, top-down, with managers imposing change and dictating the appropriate modes of behaviour required by groups and individuals within the organization. Directive change oper-ates on the premise that when groups and individuals are required to adopt different behaviours and they are exposed to the plan and rationale for the change they will develop positive attitudes towards the change and seek then to increase their relevant knowledge base. This type of change cycle invari-ably requires a hierarchical organizational structure with the emphasis on position power to operate successfully. Although the participative cycle is generally accepted as the most effective and most socially acceptable in mod-ern organizations, the directive cycle may well be appropriate and indeed welcomed by the workforce in situations of organizational crisis where staff feel more secure within the context of firm directional leadership (Fig. 4.2).

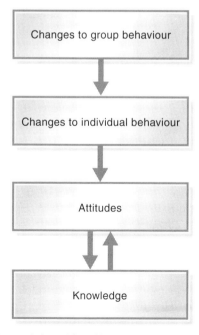

Figure 4.2 Directive change (adapted from Hersey & Blanchard 1988).

TYPES OF CHANGE: PLANNED VERSUS EMERGENT CHANGE

The literature relating to change management can present the reader with a confusing collection of strategies, models and theories as how best to manage a given change situation, so much so that complete textbooks have been devoted to the topic! However, from the wealth of literature available to us, two overall approaches are evident. These are:

- Planned change
- Emergent change.

From the titles alone the basic differences between the two approaches are evident; however, it could be useful at this point to clarify the main attributes and differences between the two approaches.

Planned change

Planned change embraces the premise that organizations can foresee and plan change in a coherent and structured way and a wide range of models and strategies are documented. These models and strategies have largely arisen from the practice of OD. OD dates back to the 1960s and was defined by Beckhard (1969), a leading proponent of the approach, as: 'An effort planned organisation-wide and managed from the top to increase organisational development and health through planned interventions in the organisation's process using behavioural science knowledge' (p. 9). More recently, French & Bell (1995) defined OD as: 'A planned and systematic process in which applied behavioural science principles and practices are introduced into ongoing organisations towards the goal of increasing individual and organisational effectiveness' (p. 1).

The key goals of OD are evident from the two definitions above, namely: individual development and organizational effectiveness. OD seeks to achieve these two goals through interventions that are systematic and planned and that utilize behavioural science knowledge and practice to the full to enhance overall organizational effectiveness and the productiveness and job satisfaction of the workforce.

Within the field of OD there are many theorists who have contributed their own models and theories (Lippett et al 1958, Bennis 1969, French & Bell 1984). However, the founding father of this approach is widely acknowledged to be Kurt Lewin. Lewin, a psychologist by background, was instrumental in describing the three step model to change management (Lewin 1947) and force field analysis (Lewin 1951), both of which have been accepted as pioneering work within the study of change management and subsequently built on by other researchers.

The three step model: unfreeze, move and refreeze

Lewin (1947) identified three stages in the change process, namely: unfreezing the current situation, moving towards the desired situation and refreezing the new situation. Unfreezing involves breaking down the normal way that people do things, disturbing old customs, beliefs and practices so that people will be prepared to accept the proposed change. This phase means continually motivating people and encouraging them to rethink the way in which they currently practise. Useful strategies for the change agent to use during this unfreezing stage is to create a feeling of dissatisfaction with the status quo and, within the context of evidence-based practice, the provision of evidence that clearly describes better outcomes for patients is a powerful motivator. Once people are motivated to change they will begin to adopt new behaviours. They will have analysed the current situation, reviewed the alternatives and decided that the best course of action is to change to the desired state. They may choose to do this through compliance with the majority decision or through deference to a management edict. Alternatively they may observe the change behaviour practised by a change agent whose expertise they respect. This invariably leads to identification with the desired behaviour which is likely to be more permanent than that achieved through compliance. The most effective means of changing behaviour and attitudes is through internalization when the individual him- or herself is the driving force to change through constantly seeking to review his or her own practice in the light of self-directed enquiry. Once the change has been introduced it is essential that it is retained and that any slippage back to the old behaviour is prevented. Individual behaviours need to be refrozen such that they then become the accepted status quo. A powerful motivator in the refreezing stage is an acceptance that the new behaviour is better than that practised previously. The change agent should seek at every opportunity to reinforce the new behaviour and to demonstrate to individuals the positive outcomes of the change. Patient satisfaction is a strong motivator in this stage.

Force field analysis

Lewin (1947) also introduced a very useful technique called force field analysis. Buchanan & Huczynski (1997) define this process as: 'A technique for assessing the factors that encourage and the factors that resist movement towards a desired target situation. Thus allowing an assessment of the viability of the change and suggesting action to alter the balance of forces, if necessary' (p. 494).

Lewin argued that all change takes place within a social field and that within every change situation it is possible to identify those factors or forces that are supporting the change (i.e. driving forces) and those that are impeding the change (i.e. restraining forces). Lewin suggested that the force

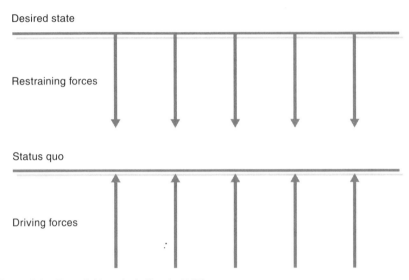

Desired state

Restraining forces

Status quo

Driving forces

Figure 4.3 Force field analysis (Lewin 1947).

exerted by the driving forces in any change situation equals that exerted by the restraining forces thus ensuring continuance of the status quo (Fig. 4.3). He postulated that to move the situation forward it was necessary to alter this balance by reducing the restraining forces and increasing the driving forces. He also suggested that it was possible to weight the strength of each driving and restraining force thus identifying the relative importance of each one. An action plan can be devised to address the identified forces with the major attention placed on reducing those restraining the change as this is likely to have the most positive effect.

It is evident that models such as force field analysis and the planned approach to change have much to offer managers and practitioners who seek to bring about change in practice situations, not least in that they provide a very comforting framework within which to work. However, there has been considerable criticism of this approach and Burns (1996) suggests that there are four major charges levelled against it. Firstly, it makes the assumption that organizations exist within a steady state that allows them to plan change strategies that will allow movement from one situation to another. Critics would suggest that organizations do not exist within a steady state but are turbulent and chaotic and it is not possible to make assumptions and action plans as things are likely to move on before they can be fully implemented. Secondly, the emphasis within planned change is on incremental and isolated change and it does not address the issue of radical and transformational change. Thirdly, it does not fully address the issue of common agreement and that not everyone is receptive to change. It makes the assumption that in all situations common agreement can be made and conflicts identified and overcome. Critics would argue that in organizations power struggles and conflicts exist that will prevent everyone signing up for the change. Finally, it makes the assumption that one model of change will suit every organization, in all situations all the time, when a more contingent approach with organizations selecting the best approach for their organization at a given point in time might be more effective.

Emergent change

The criticisms discussed above have led to a new way of thinking within the field of change management. Planned change tends to be a top-down activity with managers acting as the instigators of the change and implementing action plans whereby behaviours within the workforce are changed. Emergent change is much more of a bottom-up approach, with the change arising from practical problems which are addressed by the workforce using their own expertise to sort out solutions which are subsequently implemented and evaluated to solve the problems. Burns (1996) identifies four important aspects of consideration that need to be present within organizations if emergent change is to be facilitated effectively, namely: organizational structure, organizational culture, organizational learning and the role of management.

Organizational structure

Emergent change is most evident within organizations that support a matrix style structure, where the structure is flattened and the emphasis is on expert teams. Decision-making is devolved down to the workforce along with the resources to support locally made decisions. Communication systems are effective allowing an appropriate amount of dialogue and discussion at workforce level, which inevitably stimulates change to occur. Hierarchical structures with an emphasis on role power and where decision-making is top-down are unlikely to foster emergent change.

Organizational culture

Emergent change sits well within a culture of expertise, where the ethos of the organization is customer centred and where change is accepted as an integral component of organizational life and is to be expected and not avoided. If, as part of the evidence-based practice agenda, practitioners are required to review practice in the light of appropriate evidence and to implement changes in healthcare practice as necessary, it is very important for NHS trusts to create and support a research culture throughout the whole organization. The International Congress of Nurses (1985) identified the characteristics of an organization that is supportive of nursing research.

> **Box 4.1** Characteristics of an organizational culture that is supportive of research (International Congress of Nurses 1985)
>
> - There is flexibility in teaching, administrative and/or clinical assignments so that time for research is possible
> - Time is used for such activities as thinking about researchable questions, conducting library searches and discussion with colleagues regarding designing and carrying out a study
> - A system of formal rewards and recognition exists for persons involved in research such as promotion, salary increases and opportunities for travel
> - An informal reward system exists within the organization, i.e. peers are supportive of active (nurse) researcher's involvement and productivity in research
> - Research productivity or recognition for achievement in research is demonstrated through the numbers of grants obtained, papers presented and manuscripts published
> - There are sufficient (nurse) researchers in the organization to act as a critical mass for the development of research
> - Nurse researchers participate in multidisciplinary research projects

These characteristics are summarized in Box 4.1, and it would be valuable to assess your own organization against them.

Organizational learning

'A learning organisation is one in which people at all levels, individuals and collectively are continually increasing their capacity to produce results they really care about' (Karash 2002). A learning organization not only embraces change at all levels within the organization but seeks continually to learn as a result of the change processes. Emergent change happens within learning organizations as a result of the continual emphasis placed by the organization on developing its entire workforce to such an extent that they are 'set free' to create the kind of processes that will improve the organization's overall performance. The ethos of learning is engendered at every level within the organization and people are actively encouraged to examine their practice, to instigate change, evaluate the outcomes of the change and to learn from that change experience in order to develop a better organization.

Gerard (2002) identified eight golden rules for all learning organizations. These are presented in Box 4.2.

The role of management

The traditional view of management is that they direct and control and the workforce looks up to them for leadership and direction. For emergent change to be effective, managers need to adopt a different stance and act as facilitators and promoters of change rather than instigators and controllers. Their role is one of motivating teams to embrace and manage change by providing

---

Box 4.2   The golden rules of learning organizations (Gerard 2002)

1. **Thrive on change**
   Don't be scared of change but rather feed upon it

2. **Encourage experimentation**
   Experimentation is a necessary risk
   Encourage and reward individual initiative

3. **Communicate success and failure**
   Communicate what fails as well as what works
   Ensure the learning cycle is implemented:
   (Monitor $\rightarrow$ Review $\rightarrow$ Conclude $\rightarrow$ Change)

4. **Facilitate learning from the environment**
   Find internal and external sources of information
   Learn from your customers
   Learn from other companies

5. **Facilitate learning from employees**
   Encourage experimentation
   Invest in training
   Remove hierarchy
   Foster empowerment

6. **Reward learning**
   Boost morale with appreciation and reward
   Set benchmarks for performance appraisal

7. **Proper selfishness**
   Set clear goals and objectives

8. **Create a sense of caring**
   Care for the individual members of the organization

---

support, encouragement and the resources necessary to implement changes in practice. Managers seeking to encourage a climate of emergent change within their organizations need to be prepared to delegate responsibility and to develop their staff in order for them to cope and achieve within this devolved responsibility. The environment where emergent change is evident is also a risk environment and managers have to be prepared to live with uncertainty and ambiguity and to tolerate risk in order for improvement to take place. This is much harder for managers in service organizations such as the NHS, where mistakes can seriously affect patient safety and lead to litigation, than for managers in the production industries where mistakes may be costly but do not often have such far-reaching consequences.

SUMMARY AND CONCLUSION

In the introduction to this chapter we drew on the work of the NHS Executive (1996) and suggested that getting research/evidence-based care into practice was dependent upon three functions. The first was ensuring that all staff were made aware of the importance of practising evidence-based care and had access to the best available evidence. Providing the best possible care for all patients that is underpinned by research evidence is high on the present government's agenda. This has been demonstrated clearly in recent government reports and, to emphasize their total commitment to clinical effectiveness, the government has established NICE and CHI who will, respectively, advise and monitor the NHS. The role of the health professional in the research and development activity of the NHS has been fragmented in the past. However, with the appointment of advanced nurse practitioners and consultant nurse and therapy practitioners in most NHS trusts, and better links between trusts and universities, the NHS research and development agenda is becoming much more multiprofessional in its activity. Many researchers have described a lack of awareness of available research as being one of the reasons nurses do not implement research findings into their practice. This factor has been seriously addressed over recent years and the multiprofessional team in today's health service has access to a wide range of readily available evidence. This evidence can be obtained through books, journals, via on-line bibliographic databases and the Internet. Access to the information is not, however, the complete answer to ensuring that nurses and therapists implement research into their practice. Access needs to go hand in hand with ensuring that practitioners understand fully the evidence available. They require help to develop information technology and critical appraisal skills, preferably given by fellow practitioners skilled in this field rather than by academics in universities who may be distanced from the world of care delivery.

Secondly, it was identified that a sound understanding of how to change care in the light of research findings was essential if practitioners are to fully embrace the clinical effectiveness agenda. Readers were introduced to some of the important issues within the field of change management theory that could help to enhance their understanding of the change process and thus assist their ability to act as successful change agents in clinical practice. Key points included understanding the different levels of change and seeking to promote a bottom-up or participative approach to the change rather than the top-down directive approach which has traditionally been evident within healthcare. Bottom-up participative change actively involves the workforce at all levels and is therefore more likely to lead to a permanent internalization of the change long term. The participative approach to change is more likely to occur within an organizational structure that is matrix in style and an organizational culture that embraces expertise and devolves decision-making to the experts working in the field. In such a climate, change tends not to be planned but to emerge as a direct effect of the emphasis placed by the management on being a learning organization. Learning is the fundamental premise that underpins evidence-based practice in that practitioners employ a learning cycle in the delivery of evidenced-based care. They monitor care, they review care in the light of evidence, they make conclusions about any changes to be made that will improve care, they implement those changes and they continue to monitor them. Therefore evidence-based care will only be as good as the organization allows it to be.

REFERENCES

Bate P 1994 Strategies for cultural change. Butterworth-Heinemann, Oxford
Bate P 2001 Doing OD for a change. In: Newsletter 7 (1). Health Services Management Centre, University of Birmingham, Birmingham
Beckhard R 1969 Organisation development: strategies and models. Addison-Wesley, Reading, MA
Bennis W G 1969 Organisation development: its nature, origins and prospects. Addison-Wesley, Reading, MA
Bristol Royal Infirmary 2001 BRI inquiry final report summary. www.bristol-inquiry.org
Buchanan D, Huczynski A 1997 Organisational behaviour: an introductory text, 5th edn. Prentice Hall, London
Burns B 1996 Managing change, 2nd edn. Pitman Publishing, London
Burns T, Stalker J M 1961 The management of innovation. Tavistock, London
Closs S J, Cheater F M 1999 Evidence for nursing practice: a clarification of the issues. Journal of Advanced Nursing 30(1): 10–17
Currie L, Loftus-Hills A 2002 The nursing view of clinical governance. Nursing Standard 16(27): 40–44
Dale R, Croft A, Kenyon M 1998 Implementing clinical governance. Healthcare Quality 4(3): 22–25
Department of Health 1997 The new NHS: modern and dependable. HMSO, London
Department of Health 1998 A first class service: quality in the NHS. HMSO, London
Department of Health 1999 The Health Act. http://www.hmso.gov.uk
Department of Health 2000a The NHS plan. HMSO, London
Department of Health 2000b Shifting the balance of power. HMSO, London
DiCenso A, Cullum N, Ciliska D 1998 Implementing evidence based nursing: some misconceptions (implementing forum). Evidence Based Nursing 1: 38–40
Dunning M, Abi-Aad G, Gilbert D, Hutton H, Brown C 1999 Experience, evidence and everyday practice. King's Fund, London
Firth-Cozens J 1999 Clinical governance development needs in health service staff. British Journal of Clinical Governance 4(4): 128–134
French W L, Bell C H 1984 Organisation development. Prentice-Hall, New Jersey, USA
French W L, Bell C H 1995 Organisation development: behaviour science interventions for organisational improvement. Prentice-Hall International, New Jersey, USA
Gerard 2002 Learning organisations: golden rules. http://www.see.ed.ac.uk/~gerard/MENG/MEAB/learning_organisation/goldenrules_index…
Harvey G, Loftus-Hills A, Rycroft-Malone J et al 2002 Getting evidence into practice: the role and function of facilitation. Journal of Advanced Nursing 37(6): 577–586
Hersey P, Blanchard K 1988 Management of organizational behaviour: utilising human resources, 5th edn. Prentice-Hall, New Jersey, USA
Holt R 1999 The rhythm of quality management. British Journal of Health Care Management 5(6): 242–246
HMSO 2002 NHS Reform and Health Care Professionals Act. http://www.hmso.gov.uk
International Congress of Nurses 1985 Proceedings of assembly. RCN, London
Karash R 2002 Learning organisations. http://www.see.ed.ac.uk/~gerard/MENG/MEAB/lo_index.html
Lawrence P R, Lorsch J W 1967 Organisation and environment. Harvard Business School, Boston, USA
Lewin K 1947 Frontiers in group dynamics: concept, method and reality in social science; social equilibria and social change. Human Relations 1: 5–41
Lewin K 1951 In: Cartwright (ed) Field theory in social science. Harper and Row, New York

Lewin K 1958 Group decisions and social change. In: Swanson G E, Newcomb T M, Hartley E L (eds) Readings in social psychology. Holt, Rhinehart and Winston, New York

Lippett R, Watson J, Westley B 1958 The dynamics of planned change. Harcourt Brace and World, New York

McKenna H, Cutliffe J, McKenna P 1999 Evidence based practice: demolishing some myths. Nursing Standard 14(16): 39–42

NHS Executive 1996 Achieving effective practice: a clinical effectiveness and research information pack for nurses midwives and health visitors. Department of Health, London

Pavlov I P 1927 Conditioned reflexes [translated]. Oxford University Press, London

Preston C, Baker R 2000 Survey of the development of clinical governance in England and Wales. Journal of Clinical Governance 8(3): 118–123

Rodgers S 1994 An exploratory study of research utilization by nurses in general medical and surgical wards. Journal of Advanced Nursing 20: 904–911

Thompson C, McCaughan D, Cullum N, Sheldon T A, Mulhall A, Thompson D R 2001 The accessibility of research-based knowledge for nurses in United Kingdom acute care settings. Journal of Advanced Nursing 36(1): 11–22

Walshe K, Freeman T, Latham L, Wallace L, Spurgeon P 2000 Clinical governance: from policy to practice. Health Services Management Centre, School of Public Policy, University of Birmingham, Birmingham

York University 1999 Centre for Reviews and Dissemination, effectiveness bulletin. York University, York

5

Research for practice

Ros Carnwell

Editors' comment

This chapter explores, from the perspective of a number of healthcare initiatives today, some aspects of research that are often overlooked in standard research texts. Following a contextual review, consideration is given to three approaches to research that may be utilized in clinical areas to evaluate practice. They include action research, critical theory and evaluation research. The chapter's main focus is on using research to bring about changes in practice, rather than as an enterprise in itself. The author argues that qualitative research approaches are more effective at achieving this.

INTRODUCTION

Preference of for EBP

Within two dominant research paradigms commonly used in healthcare – qualitative/interpretative and quantitative/positivist – there is an array research approaches that are relevant to healthcare practitioners. The often an assumption within healthcare, however, that the most reliable research evidence on which to base healthcare practices comes from a positivist perspective, specifically experimental research such as randomized control trials or from large-scale quantitative surveys. While this assumption is laudable, recent changes in healthcare delivery have set the scene for the use of more practice-orientated research approaches. The recent focus on evidence-based practice requires treatment decisions to be based on a variety of evidence including research, but also, and importantly, from patients' preferences and the expert opinion of experienced professionals.

The importance of the patient/client or 'user perspective' is also acknowledged within the national service frameworks (Department of Health 1997), which require patients to be given information about what they can expect from the health service. This change in thinking, together with a need for quality improvement (Department of Health 1999), provides the scope for use of a wide range of research approaches. Contemporary research approaches, rather than requiring objectivity and distance between the researcher and subjects, celebrate the close proximity of the researcher to participants being studied and it is this proximity that brings researchers close to practice.

This chapter will begin by exploring some recent developments that have impacted on the need for a strong research base in healthcare. It will consider issues arising from these changes and practical examples of research that could be conducted will be highlighted. The chapter will then return to these practical examples to consider approaches to research and methods of data collection that could be used to address them. The emphasis will be on 'research and practice' and the examples will reflect this emphasis.

A chapter of this length will not be able to explore the whole range of research approaches but this is not problematic as there are numerous research texts that do that. Rather, three research approaches have been selected for further discussion because of their relevance to contemporary healthcare practice. These are: action research, evaluation research, and critical research methods.

RECENT DEVELOPMENTS IN PRACTICE AND THEIR IMPACT ON RESEARCH

The National Health Service (NHS) plan (Department of Health 2000) has proposed closer working relationships between health and social care workers, requiring healthcare staff to extend their roles and use a wider range of skills. Furthermore, patients and clients are being given a real say in how care is provided, with patient advocates, patients' surveys and forums being established to ensure this becomes a reality. These changes are a driving force behind the need for research in healthcare. The contemporary NHS requires evidence from trust and health authority managers of the value of any changes that have taken place. The skills of research and knowledge of research approaches are therefore essential in providing evidence of the impact of new developments, including cost-effectiveness, in healthcare delivery.

These changes not only impact upon accountability of health professionals, but also affect the way in which services are delivered to clients and patients. As a result of the NHS and Community Care Act (Department of Health 1990), for example, many 'technologically dependent' patients are now cared for in their own homes, thus reducing the risk of them losing their independence (King's Fund 1994). This change sets the scene for further changes in the delivery of primary care services, with more work and power transferred to GPs (NHSE 1997). Indeed, primary care services are set to change still further as a result of the NHS plan. *Primary Care, General Practice and the NHS Plan* (Department of Health 2001), for example, states that: 'patients will be seen more quickly in modern premises, by GPs less burdened by bureaucracy and with more time for each patient they see'.

One of the disciplines to be affected by these changes is the community children's nurse, whose expert knowledge has been transferred to the community setting, where children's nurses teach and support parents through the trauma of caring for an ill child. At least two studies have revealed a patient/child preference for being cared for at home with professional support, rather than in hospital (Balling & McCubbin 2001, Sartain et al 2001), while a further study identifies the dilemmas and problems in providing home-based respite support to parents of young children with complex healthcare needs (Olsen & Maslin-Prothero 2001). Evaluating the effectiveness of this new type of service delivery might include research into how well parents are prepared for the discharge of their children from hospital, the education and training needs of community children's nurses and an evaluation of the additional financial burden on parents who might have to give up work to care for their child.

Parallel to these changes in the nature of service delivery, other changes also have the potential to change the face of healthcare. Two such changes are the development of specialist, advanced and consultant practitioners and integrated healthcare teams.

During the 1990s political and professional debates about the scope of nursing roles led to nurses, midwives and health visitors developing their scope and levels of practice (Ashburner et al 1997, Department of Health 2000, Frost 1998, Wilson-Barnett et al 2000). The PREP recommendations (UKCC 1990) led to the creation of specialist and advanced nursing practice, to which were added consultant practitioners as a result of the NHS Plan (Department of Health 2000). Specialist practice degree level qualifications now allow nurses to build on specialist expertise gained following diploma level education. Advanced practitioners in nursing and allied health professions are educated at masters degree level. Advanced practitioners work in either primary or secondary care as autonomous practitioners, using expert skills in holistic health assessment as well as research skills to challenge the boundaries of practice. The development of these roles has evolved from a need to provide quality care for patients and clients (Snyder & Mirr 1995) as well as being driven by economic policy which controls escalating costs rather than advances in practice (Elcock 1996). Specialist, advanced and consultant practitioner roles are in their infancy in the UK, although a number of studies have evaluated advanced nurse practitioner roles in North America (Office of Technology Assessment 1986, Mirr 1995, Mundinger et al 2000) and UK studies are beginning to emerge (Kinnersley et al 2000, Venning et al 2000, Daly & Carnwell 2003). More research will need to be carried out to evaluate their effectiveness, but in the meantime debate is ongoing with the regulatory bodies about ensuring that the evolution of new titles is accompanied by appropriate levels of competence and associated professional registration (Nursing Midwifery Council 2003).

Questions that could be asked of each type of practice relate to professional differences, asking, for example, is the care provided by an advanced or consultant nurse practitioner comparable to that provided by a GP? This may link to cost-effectiveness. For example: do the gains resulting from employing practitioners with first degree and masters or doctoral degree level education outweigh the costs of their education?

Integrated healthcare teams are another change in primary healthcare which need to be researched in order to monitor their effectiveness. Primary healthcare teams, as originally established, functioned with team members having little knowledge of colleagues' skills or responsibilities, thus resulting in duplication of roles (Baileff 2000). The need for more effective teamwork was mentioned in numerous government reforms during the 1990s (e.g. Department of Health 1993a, 1997, 1998), but it was the Department of Health (1999) *Making a Difference* report that emphasized most fervently the need for teamwork within healthcare in order to bring about the proposed government reforms. This was reiterated in *Making a Difference: Integrated Working in Primary Care* (Department of Health 2000), which required nurses to pool their skills in order to meet the needs of the population.

Integrated healthcare teams involve a team of healthcare staff with differing expertise drawing upon and sharing each other's roles, resulting in more effective team working and collaboration (Rink et al 2000) and ensuring that services are developed based upon need (Adams & Thomas 2001). Rather than each healthcare discipline, such as district nursing, health visiting and practice nursing, working independently, they each perform some of the roles of the others, while also drawing on the specialist expertise of colleagues when necessary. Obviously, staff operating in integrated healthcare teams need to be trained in procedures in which they have been previously unfamiliar, and this has important implications for professional development. The additional expertise of nurses, however, ensures that patients experience improved care based upon evidence, together with a more flexible and accessible service (Forrester & Kline 1997). Researching the effectiveness of this type of change might therefore involve asking questions such as: How can the present primary care team become integrated so that care can be delivered more effectively? What beneficial influences does integrated healthcare teamwork have on working practices in primary care? Alternatively, what impact has the integrated healthcare team had on the uptake of primary care services?

Another important change affecting healthcare is clinical supervision, which was one of the twelve targets in *A Vision for the Future* (Department of Health 1993b). Clinical supervision involves an interaction between two or more practitioners within a safe environment, which facilitates reflective critical analysis of care, thus enhancing the quality of services provided (Bishop 1997). The requirement to review the practice of individuals and the quality of their services as a result of clinical governance provides an incentive for the embedding of clinical supervision across a wide range of practice settings (Butterworth & Woods 1999). However, although professions such as psychotherapy (Kagan & Werner 1977) and social work (Kadushin 1985) have long embraced this philosophy, clinical supervision in nursing has only developed during the past decade (Johns 1993, Faugier & Butterworth 1994, Fowler 1996, Bishop 1997, Bond & Holland 1998).

Present trends in clinical supervision include: concerns about increased accountability; the demand to improve standards of care; and increased emphasis on reflective practice and lifelong learning (Bond & Holland 1998). There has been considerable research into clinical supervision, especially in nursing (e.g. Malin 2000, Milne & Oliver 2000, Veeramah 2002), with fewer examples in allied health professions (e.g. Weaver 2001), while in medical education clinical supervision is the subject of very little research and development (Kilminster & Jolly 2000). One research question worthy of consideration would be therefore: What would be the benefits of clinical supervision in medical education?

The changes to healthcare so far discussed raise many research questions and changes in future will contribute further to the need for research. The effects of these changes are yet to be seen, but any changes in quality of patient care will need to be monitored carefully. Now that some changes affecting healthcare staff have been identified, the next section of this chapter will consider some appropriate research methods to address these issues.

USING RESEARCH IN PRACTICE

This section will use some of the examples of practice discussed above to demonstrate the type of research methodologies that might be employed most usefully in healthcare research. Having a firm evidence base to inform practice also requires that research methods are appropriate to healthcare problems and that they will provide solutions that healthcare staff can use in practice. Three approaches to research will be explored in this chapter: action research, evaluation research, and critical research methods.

Action research

Action research, as the name suggests, is concerned with bringing about action (through change) as a result of the research process. The originator of the term is Kurt Lewin, a German social psychologist who worked in the USA in the late 1930s where his research focused on education and problems in minority groups, as well as racism and fascism. Lewin was interested in helping people to see things in a new way, which he believed was more likely to be successful with groups than with individuals because people are more likely to commit themselves to change when it is made in a group context.

Lewin's (1947a) system of action research was thus created with the purpose not only of bringing about change (see Ch. 4) but also measuring change to demonstrate that it had occurred. The existing situation, therefore, had to be studied first, then the event would take place, following which the situation would be studied again to see what changes had taken place. Any changes to the situation could then be argued to have resulted from the event because the situation had been thoroughly studied beforehand.

Lewin went on to propose that action research is a spiral of circular activities with a series of steps, each step influencing the next. Thus an action research project involves a preparatory stage, followed by a series of steps, each of which is influenced by the one before. The preparatory stage of the action research cycle is crucial since it involves fact-finding to establish the context and history of the idea being researched. This stage needs to involve all people involved in the system in which the research is to take place. Facts also need to be fed back to this group as part of the cycles of the research. Once the fact-finding is complete and the group has a thorough understanding of the current situation, a general plan can be formed.

Putting the general plan into action is the next stage in the cycle, and in developing an action plan the researchers are assuming that the situation can be improved. This involves a series of action steps, each of which involves the same four stages: planning, acting, observing and reflecting (Lewin 1947b). When Lewin proposed his theory of action research, it was usual for expert researchers to enter organizations and to seek permission to test out their theories of human behaviour and to bring about change. Present day use of action research is somewhat different. It is more usual for staff such as health professionals to recognize that change is necessary and could be brought about by action research, and then to seek the advice of expert action researchers on how to design the study.

A contemporary interpretation of Lewin's framework is produced by Burns (2000, pp. 444–445), who suggests a model involving the following seven sub-stages (adapted from Burns 2000):

1. Identification, evaluation and formulation of the problem
2. Fact-finding in order to fully describe the problem
3. Review of research literature in order to learn from comparable studies
4. Having generated hypotheses, gather information relevant to testing them
5. Select research procedures and materials and negotiate proposed actions with stakeholders
6. Implement action plan, including: methods of data collection and keeping of reports, monitoring of tasks, feedback to research team, classification and analysis of data and evaluation strategy
7. Interpretation of data and overall evaluation of the project, by production of case study report at the end of each cycle.

Using the above framework, an action research project could be used to develop the integrated healthcare team referred to above.

Stage one could involve a clear formulation of the problem, for example in terms of the following questions:

- How can the present primary care team become integrated so that care can be delivered more effectively?
- Which members of the team should become part of the integrated care team and which members should continue to practise independently of the integrated team?
- How should the integrated team be managed?

Stage two, the fact-finding stage, would involve all team members analysing the situation and describing the specific problems and how they would expect these to be overcome by implementing the integrated team. Problems might include, for example, duplication of roles, deskilling of staff if they practise certain skills infrequently, and delay in delivery of services if staff with appropriate skills are not available when needed. These observations would then be compared with current literature on integrated primary care teams, in *stage three*. These would provide a clear understanding of the problem, from which some hypotheses might be generated such as: 'integrated primary care teams reduce patient/client waiting times in GP surgeries' or 'patients will be more satisfied with services provided by an integrated primary care, than with the existing team'.

During *stage four*, evidence would be gathered that the selected hypotheses are realistic. Burns (2000) points out that this does not mean that they should be tested statistically, since in action research hypotheses are more tentative than would be found in quantitative research. Gathering of evidence may result in other explanations for the situation, for example the team might question whether a reduction in waiting times might occur due to other reasons, such as the employment of additional staff.

It is during *stage five* that the more precise nature of the research would be developed. Responsibilities of different staff members would be an important part of this stage. Different members of the research team would take responsibility for managing different components of the project. In this respect, some members of the project team might also be members of the integrated primary care team. This demonstrates the collaborative nature of action research, which, although very positive, can potentially result in bias in data collection. Responsibilities would therefore need to be allocated judiciously to avoid staff collecting and interpreting data that was closely related to their own practice. Typical data collected would include: waiting times, patient throughput, patient satisfaction, and frequency of use of skills by different staff. Such data could be collected by a range of instruments such as diaries, interviews, focus groups and questionnaires, all of which would be negotiated during this important stage of the cycle. Negotiation with stakeholders would also include permission from the primary care team to collect data and to visit the practice during specified times. The research team would also negotiate specific details of the project such as: storage and analysis of questionnaires, interviews and diaries; frequency of reports and members of the research team responsible for their production; and allocation of responsibility for monitoring that all data had been completed at the agreed points.

With such precision in stage five, *stage six* becomes straightforward and involves each member of the team implementing their particular tasks. During this stage, the monitoring of data collection would be discussed at frequent meetings of the research team and findings would be shared with stakeholders. This stage leads naturally to the final stage, *stage seven*, in which the data are interpreted and a case study report is produced. A case study report of the outcomes of the first cycle could, for example, be presented to the primary care team, during which preparation for the second cycle of the research could be discussed. This would involve a repetition of the first step of identifying and formulating problems that would have arisen out of the findings of the first cycle.

This example illustrates the collaborative nature of contemporary approaches to action research. It also exemplifies all seven characteristics of action research identified by Hart & Bond (1995). Hart & Bond argue that these seven characteristics distinguish action research from other methodologies in that action research is: educative; deals with individuals as members of a group; is problem-focused, context-specific and future orientated; involves a change intervention; aims at improvement and involvement; involves a cyclic process in which research, action and evaluation are interlinked, and is founded on a research relationship in which those involved are participants in the change process. It is important to note, however, that practitioners involved may play the 'action research game' in which they cooperate during the research but then fail to play by the rules once the project has been completed (Grundy 1982). As Grundy (1982) points out, this is more likely to occur in projects where the practitioners were not sufficiently involved in developing the project in the first place and were not committed to the ideas that were driving the project forward.

A type of action research that is often more challenging occurs when changes need to be brought about, but certain obstacles, such as bureaucratic or managerial practices, prevent the possibility of change ever taking place. Action research in this context will be discussed later in this chapter when critical research methods are discussed.

Collecting data in action research

Action research carried out in healthcare settings commonly uses focus group interviews as a method of collecting data. Using action research to evaluate changes resulting from integrated healthcare teams would be amenable to this approach. Groups of between six and ten members are normally sufficient, and therefore the whole team would be divided into groups. The groups would be multidisciplinary in nature so that the different perspectives of each discipline could be represented at each interview. Each interview should be taped and transcribed. The main decisions made by each group should then be fed back to members of the other groups, thus feeding back into the action research cycle, so that future decisions can be made on the basis of the views of all members. Another method of collecting data frequently used in action research is the use of SWOT analysis. Team members would be asked to identify all the *s*trengths, *w*eaknesses, *o*pportunities and *t*hreats that had occurred as a result of working as an integrated team. Members could then discuss and agree methods of exploiting existing strengths and opportunities, while considering ways of overcoming existing weaknesses and threats.

Getting research into practice using action research

The dynamic nature of action research makes this research approach an excellent example of how research can change practice. Lewin's original proposal of using research to initiate change could be viewed as an early attempt to get research into practice. Contemporary use of action research has gone further still, with emphasis on using practitioners as collaborators *in* research rather than bringing in experts to conduct action research *on* the organization. The practical nature of action research also makes it acceptable to health professionals.

Evaluation research

Evaluation research shares some similarities with action research in that it is concerned with existing programmes and practice. Whereas action research always seeks to use the research process to bring about change, evaluation research seeks to use the research process to determine the value of a programme. A comprehensive definition of evaluation is provided by Patton (1997, p. 23) as follows: 'Programme evaluation is the systematic collection of information about the activities, characteristics, and outcomes of programs to make judgments about the program, improve program effectiveness, and/or inform decisions about future programming.' Patton also draws an interesting distinction between programme evaluation and research. Whereas research is undertaken to uncover new knowledge, test theories, establish truth and make generalizations to other settings, programme evaluation attempts to inform decisions and clarify options, and is therefore more action than theory orientated.

Evaluation research has grown out of different disciplines, such as medicine, epidemiology, statistics, and social science (Øvretveit 2000), and this has resulted in evaluators having to make difficult decisions at the paradigm

Table 5.1 Approaches to evaluation research

	Purpose	Focus
Goal-orientated	To measure the extent to which the programme had achieved its intended goals	Goals must be precise and measurable, enabling evaluator to design instruments to effectively measure achievement of goals
Goal-free (Scriven 1972)	To focus on unintended consequences	Needs-based approach in which the evaluator focuses on what needs the programme is meeting
Illuminative evaluation (Parlett & Hamilton (1976))	To describe and interpret innovatory programmes, how they operate, their advantages/disadvantages – thus illuminating complex questions	Is based in anthropological paradigm, and might use ethnographic interviews to collect data
Patton's (1997) approaches:		
• Decision-focused approach	To provide the right information at the right time to help the decision-makers to make the right decisions	Evaluator works closely with decision-makers to find out what type of information they need from the organization to enable them to make their decisions
• Utilization-focused	To design evaluation studies with careful consideration of how everything that is done within the project will be used	Evaluator works closely with intended users to help them to decide what type of evaluation they need, including the design of questions about what needs to be answered
Four approaches (Øvretveit 2000):		
• Experimental	To seek evidence of *effect* and *causes*	*Outcomes* by testing *hypotheses*
• Economic	To calculate *resources used* and *benefits*	Inputs, activity and outputs by using *outcomes measurements*
• Developmental	To help providers to *improve* in the *short term*	Process using *qualitative* methods
• Managerial	*Accountability* and *performance management*	Inputs, processes and outputs, using *both qualitative and quantitative methods*

Five forms (Owen & Rogers 1999):

• Proactive evaluation	To assist stakeholders in making decisions on development of the programme *before* it is designed	Needs assessment, research review, and review of best practice and creation of benchmarks
• Clarificatory evaluation	To clarify the internal structure and functioning of a programme for stakeholders, who may need advice about how best to implement the programme	Programme logic development, involving interviews of programme staff and development of a map of what the programme is supposed to do; and accreditation of the worth of the programme guidelines
• Interactive evaluation	To use findings to facilitate learning and decision-making by stakeholders	Responsive evaluation in order to take into account perspectives of different stakeholders; of action research; quality review or institutional self-study; developmental evaluation involving continuous improvement; and empowerment evaluation to assist participants to evaluate their own programmes
• Monitoring evaluation	To evaluate established programmes to ascertain success or otherwise	Component analysis, devolved performance assessment and systems analysis in order to indicate performance against an agreed standard
• Impact evaluation	To evaluate outcomes of an established programme	*Objectives-based*, process-outcomes studies, needs-based evaluation, goal-free evaluation, performance audit

level (Clarke & Dawson 1999). Moreover, depending on their philosophical stance, evaluators often disagree about such issues as the role of the researcher, the questions the researcher should ask, and the best methods to use (Øvretveit 2000). Clarke & Dawson further point out that although evaluation was initially dominated by the natural science paradigm with its emphasis on quantitative measurement, experiments and hypothesis testing, recent critics have argued that, while it is possible to determine whether a programme has had an impact, 'they offer little insight into the social processes which actually account for the change being observed' (p. 55). However, Clarke & Dawson also draw attention to the fact that by depicting the two methodologically distinct paradigms as incompatible, purists risk actively discouraging multi-method designs.

Numerous authors have attempted to make sense of evaluative research by categorizing the possible approaches used. Examples of some authors' approaches are presented in Table 5.1.

Although contemporary evaluations use a variety of research approaches, before the last two decades evaluation studies were much less eclectic. Traditionally, evaluations were goal-orientated in their approach and evaluators would measure the extent to which the programme had achieved its intended goals. Goals, therefore, needed to be precise and measurable, and the evaluator's task would be to design instruments that would effectively measure the achievement of objectives. Indeed, Patton (1997) argues that the evaluator should be involved in the development of goals from the outset in order to ensure that they are amenable to evaluation. Typically, in healthcare settings, specific treatment interventions were applied and the effects would be measured both before and after treatment. The quantitative paradigm would be the one of choice and instrument design, sampling and statistical testing were crucial to the success of the evaluation.

Returning to the practice examples identified earlier, the goal-orientated approach can be illustrated using the example of an advanced nurse practitioner who runs a nurse-led pain management clinic and decides to evaluate the effectiveness of the services she provides. Although she could do this by sending questionnaires to all her patients asking them how satisfied they were with the treatment they had received, patients might express satisfaction with any service, regardless of whether it had been effective, just because they were grateful that they had been seen by a health professional. An alternative would be to define the intended outcomes of the service she is providing from the outset. One intended outcome could be 'for each patient to experience a minimum of 50% pain relief after one month of treatment'. This is precise and measurable. She could develop a pain scale from 1 to 10 and ask the patients to indicate their level of pain on the scale before treatment. She could then prescribe the appropriate intervention and use the same measuring instrument at the end of one month. Naturally, she would not be satisfied with the response of just one patient, and could not be sure that the patients would not have made the same improvements by using the usual treatments prescribed by a GP. Ideally, she would need to randomly assign patients to either an intervention group, or a control group, and would need a large enough sample, at least 30 in each group (Hicks 1990), for the results to have any statistical significance. This demonstrates how the goal-orientated approach is traditionally experimental in nature. Traditionally such experiments would have been conducted as part of large-scale evaluations, carried out by expert evaluators who would produce a summative report at the end of the evaluation study. Expert evaluators would also be important to avoid any bias that might arise by a member of staff collecting data relating to their own practice. In the above example, patients might feel obliged to say that their pain had reduced if the nurse who had provided the pain relief was collecting data and this would clearly bias the results.

This example indicates some important points about goal-orientated evaluations. First, the goals must be clearly stated at the beginning, and it is useful to seek the advice of an evaluator at this stage. Second, it is best to avoid the potential bias arising from evaluating one's own practice, by charging an independent person with collecting the data. Third, the goal-orientated approach lends itself to experimental methods and use of the quantitative approach to data collection. The goal-orientated approach typifies the emphasis on the quantitative paradigm in early evaluations. According to Patton (1997, pp. 272–273), by the late 1970s 'the evaluation profession had before it the broad outlines of two competing research paradigms' which he refers to as the qualitative/naturalistic and quantitative/experimental paradigms. Table 5.1 exemplifies the eclectic mix of approaches facing the contemporary evaluator, an early example being the goal-free approach.

Scriven (1972) suggests that the goal-free approach assumes that by focusing exclusively on goals (as in the goal-orientated approach), important unintended consequences of the programme might be missed. Hence, Scriven likens the goal-free approach to a needs-based approach in which the evaluator focuses on what needs the programme is meeting. Using this approach, the programme might be seen to fall short of its intended goals, but could still be seen as successful in meeting local needs. Using this approach, our advanced nurse practitioner might not be so concerned about the effectiveness of her pain management clinic and whether it achieved its intended outcomes. Rather, she would need to look wider to assess her patients' needs, and to evaluate the extent that patients felt their needs had been met through attending the clinic. Patients' needs might be expressed in terms of valuing opportunities to discuss their pain and how it affects various aspects of their life, and this might be as important to some patients as the pain relief itself. Discovering unintended consequences of a programme can be just as important as demonstrating the achievement of its goals. A strategy such as this, however, means that the researcher is close to the participants, often acquiring data through interviewing. The potential for bias is even greater and it would be unwise therefore for the advanced nurse practitioner, in this case, to collect the data her/himself.

Not too dissimilar to the goal-free approach is illuminative evaluation (Parlett & Hamilton 1976). Although originally designed for schools, the descriptive, exploratory nature of illuminative evaluation is appropriate for healthcare settings. The evaluation of the care of technologically dependent children in the home would lend itself to this approach. This could include ethnographic interviews of parents to elicit their experiences and concerns relating to caring for their children at home. This would include an evaluation of what the parents consider to be the significant features of the programme and the critical processes involved (Parlett & Hamilton 1976). This would then produce an account of any emerging problems and how they could be solved.

The example of technologically dependent children would also be amenable to the decision-focused approach to evaluation. The decisions are important in this approach, rather than the people who make them, with the evaluator assisting decision-makers to make the right decisions, by providing the right information at the right time (Patton 1997). The development of a hospital-at-home scheme in providing seamless care would be a good example of how this might take place. Hospital and community managers would need to negotiate how services from hospital could be transferred to the community, how technological equipment would be maintained and how staff would be prepared for their new role. They could plan and implement all of this without the help of an evaluator, but if they did so, they would have no formal way of knowing whether their proposals had been effective. By involving an evaluator at every stage of the decision-making process, they would be given the best information to enable them to make the best decisions. The evaluator could, for example, interview staff about their hopes and fears in relation to working in the community and what additional training they might need. Data might also be collected on the availability of non-human resources in the community, and the finances required for extra equipment. Although the decision-focused approach sounds like a useful way of helping managers to make appropriate decisions, it does also have its critics. Important decisions are not always made in the boardroom, and therefore the evaluator might not always be able to provide the right information at the right time. Furthermore, as Patton (1997) points out, people who make decisions do so incrementally over a long period of time, rather than at a predetermined moment. Moreover, people also have their idiosyncrasies and therefore the subjective whim of an individual, rather than information collected by an evaluator, might influence an important decision.

A suggested approach proposed by Patton (1997) to overcome the problems of the above approach is utilization-focused evaluation, which he defines as being 'done for and with specific, intended primary users for specific, intended uses' (Patton 1997). Utilization-focused evaluation is concerned with designing evaluation studies with careful consideration of how everything that is done within the project will be used. This requires that the evaluator works closely with intended users to help them to decide what type of evaluation they need. The first step of this process is to help intended users to define their own questions that they want answering about their own programme.

Returning to the practice examples at the beginning of this chapter, it is possible to see how the implementation and evaluation of clinical supervision might raise several questions amenable to this approach. Utilization-focused evaluation would involve all users, including different grades of staff. Consequently, supervisors and supervisees would work together to frame the questions to which they wanted answers. For example, managers might ask the question: 'How effective is clinical supervision in identifying training needs of staff?' A clinical supervisor might ask: 'What impact has clinical supervision had on enabling staff to deal with stressful situations that occur in practice?' And a supervisee might want to ask: 'What will be the potential benefits of clinical supervision in enabling junior staff to enhance their career prospects?'

Research questions concerning clinical supervision could also be addressed, however, using other contemporary approaches to evaluation research. For example, 'What would be the benefits of clinical supervision in medical education?' could be addressed using Øvretveit's (2000) economic approach. This would involve the evaluator calculating the resources used and benefits arising from them. This would require collecting data relating to: resources (inputs), such as training of supervisors and supervisor and supervisee time used in clinical supervision; activity, such as the nature and number of clinical supervision sessions convened; and outputs, such as the impact of clinical supervision on the delivery of medical education. Equally, Øvretveit's (2000) developmental approach could also be used for this research problem as it is concerned with helping stakeholders – in this case participants in medical education – to develop and improve their performance through the support of the evaluator.

The role of the researcher is important in any research and it is interesting that the researcher's role differs considerably depending upon the type of evaluation approach used. In both experimental and economic approaches (Øvretveit 2000) the researcher is detached and scientific, as befits the use of quantitative research. Researchers using the developmental approach, although independent of the programme being evaluated, could have a similar relationship to the stakeholders that action researchers adopt, that is, they can adopt a collaborative relationship with stakeholders, such as service managers and other people working in the service. Researchers using a managerial approach, on the other hand, are likely to adopt an inspectorial, detached role.

Another research question posed in the above discussion related to integrated healthcare teams was: 'What beneficial influences does integrated healthcare teamwork have on working practices in primary care?' This question would be amenable to three of the approaches suggested by Owen & Rogers (1999): interactive evaluation, monitoring evaluation, and impact evaluation. Interactive evaluation would facilitate learning and decision-making by stakeholders. The evaluator would be interested in gaining information from all people who had a stake in the programme, such as all members of the primary care team, as well as receptionists and the practice manager. Working collaboratively with the practice would enable the evaluator to facilitate their reflection on the improvements to their working practices. This would result in continuous improvement as a result of being involved in the research and thereby gaining deeper understanding of practices. Monitoring evaluation can only be used to assess the effectiveness of an established programme. In this case an agreed standard would already have been set. An example of possible agreed standards could be that:

- All patients have been treated by a healthcare practitioner within 20 minutes of entering the GP practice
- Each member of the integrated team has a broader repertoire of skills
- Patients express satisfaction with services used
- Staff express a high degree of job satisfaction.

The different components of the programme (the integrated team) would then be analysed to discover whether the agreed standards had been achieved. A skills analysis conducted both before and after the development of the integrated team, for example, would reveal whether the repertoire of skills of each team member had increased. A similar process would be used for an impact evaluation, although this type of evaluation would also be interested in unintended consequences of the programme. An example could be that staff members report less stress, and greater involvement of initiatives outside of the practice, such as membership of primary care trusts. These examples demonstrate the potential of evaluation research to draw on a wide range of research methods, according to the research problem. What is particularly interesting is the proximity of contemporary evaluation research methods to practice.

Collecting data in evaluation research

Patton (1997) provides an excellent synopsis of the major emphases adopted by different approaches to evaluation. He begins with the original thesis that underpinned the goal-orientated approach, that is, that the evaluator would carry out objective, scientific experiments to collect quantitative data. Hypotheses would be tested, theories would be validated, statistics would be used to analyse data, and generalizations would be made. Our nurse-led pain clinic would exemplify this approach. Patton contrasts this with what he terms an 'antithesis' in which exploratory research is carried out using naturalistic methods to look for qualitative differences. The evaluator would use a subjective stance and would be closely involved with the participants under study, as in the example of our nurse practitioner using a goal-free approach, or the illuminative evaluation approach to evaluate the care given to technologically dependent children in the home. Analysis would be qualitative including content analysis and grounded theory. Patton favours the use of a synthesis of these different paradigms. In focusing on intended users he argues for combining both qualitative and quantitative methods as befits the questions raised by various stakeholders in the programme.

Getting research into practice using evaluation research

The value of evaluation research in getting research into practice can be summed up in the words of Patton (1997, p. 4), who states that:

How evaluations are used affects the spending of billions of dollars to fight problems of poverty, disease, ignorance, joblessness, mental anguish, crime, hunger and inequality. How are programs that combat these societal ills to be judged? How does one distinguish effective from ineffective programs? And how can evaluations be conducted in ways that lead to use? How do we avoid producing reports that gather dust on bookshelves, unread and unused?

Patton's concerns mirror the need to evaluate health service initiatives, to distinguish good practices from bad practices so that services can be improved. Such an approach to research is compatible with an age of quality assurance, accountability and the need to measure outcomes. By focusing on the utility value of evaluation, Patton attempts to narrow the gap between 'generating evaluation findings and actually using those findings for program decision-making and improvement' (p. 6).

Critical research methods

Of the three research approaches discussed in this chapter, critical research methods are arguably the most qualitative in orientation, while also being most closely allied to practice and research participants. Critical research methods are based on critical theory, which includes neo-Marxism, feminism, materialism and participatory inquiry (Guba & Lincoln 1994). Rather than pinpointing and recording fine details within the research process, critical theory recognizes that certain social phenomena deserve examination due to an interest in emancipation of participants (Alvesson & Sköldberg 2001). According to Alvesson & Sköldberg (2001), typical research questions are those that certain élite groups are reluctant to have answered, but ones which might be crucial to a disadvantaged group. Alvesson & Sköldberg provide an interesting contrast to evaluation research questions, drawing on an example from Perrow (1978), who, rather than asking 'How can we do more to achieve our goals?' asked 'What actually drives these operations?' Underpinning this alternative approach is a view that stated goals are driven by external functions, such as the interest of leaders, rather than the needs of clients.

One type of critical research is critical ethnography (Thomas 1993), which assumes that cultural forces shape the social conditions that disadvantage some groups more than others. Moreover, institutions of power limit choices, confer legitimacy and guide our daily routine (Boudieu 1991, Thomas 1993). The ontological assumption is that there is something else there that will take us beneath the surface world of accepted appearances to reveal the darker, oppressive side of social life (Thomas 1993). The purpose of critical ethnography is to reveal the politics of the multilayered complexity of communication (Forester 1992). Critical ethnography as a research approach moves beyond the philosophical debate which seems to surround critical research. The critical component focuses on the relations of power and how they are exhibited in society, while the ethnographic component is both empirical and sensitive to socially constructed meanings and how they can be uncovered (Giddens 1984, Marcus 1986). Thus, critical ethnography involves using knowledge for social change and emancipation.

These beliefs suggest that life experiences are shaped by social, political, cultural, economic, ethnic and gender values, and that this occurs over generations. This fundamental belief has considerable impact on the way research is carried out. Critical researchers argue that scientific methods are inappropriate to discover the truth, because the nature of social injustice makes truth value-laden. Critical research, therefore, focuses on values held by society and how these result in social injustice that affects people's lives. Research focusing on people's lives will by necessity use qualitative methods. The researcher enters into a dialogue with the participants, often through interviewing and attempts to uncover experiences of struggle and conflict. Typical social injustices that would be brought into the open through critical research would be the experiences of different types of inequality, such as racial or sexual inequality, or inequalities in health arising from social class. However, the critical researcher does not stop at bringing these social injustices into the open. Critical research is both participatory and emancipatory. This means that the people being studied will participate in the research process themselves, and through this process will become emancipated so that they can take control over their own situation.

Collecting data using critical research methods

Returning again to the practical examples earlier in this chapter, it is possible to see how certain research problems and research questions lend themselves to critical research methods. The transfer of secondary care to the primary care sector could further disadvantage people who already have few facilities at their disposal. Using quantitative methods such as questionnaire surveys would not really give vulnerable people a voice. However, the researcher who becomes genuinely involved with participants through interviewing and observations, helping them to make their views known through advocacy and empowerment, will help vulnerable groups to take control over their own lives and the services offered to them, thus changing things for the better. A typical example of this would be a practitioner working with people with mental health problems and, through understanding gained from interviewing, helping them to acquire appropriate accommodation and support services so that they could live independently in the community.

Critical research methods can also involve a variety of different approaches to research. Action research is just one example of how an approach to research can be used from different perspectives, a critical perspective being just one way of conducting action research. As indicated earlier, action research might employ a critical perspective when certain obstacles prevent the possibility of change taking place (Grundy 1982). In such circumstances, the action steps would need to involve some level of emancipation in order for change to take place. Only when people are sufficiently emancipated can they overcome obstacles that have been put in their way. Two examples from the earlier discussion will serve to illustrate this point: healthcare for technologically dependent children at home, and implementing clinical supervision in advanced healthcare practice.

Caring for technologically dependent children at home will create tremendous strain for parents. They might have to overcome various obstacles such as fear of using complicated technological equipment and anxiety associated with the well-being of their child. Children's nurses could work with parents during the fact-finding stage to discover the main problems and concerns associated with nursing technologically dependent children at home. Working with parents, they could then work through the action stages to develop an action plan, which together they would implement, observe and reflect upon. The purpose behind using a critical research perspective in this scenario would be to emancipate the parents to bring about the change process themselves so that they would be better equipped to care for their child.

The second example to illustrate this approach is the implementation of clinical supervision by advanced nurse practitioners in primary care. Morrow (1994) makes the point that 'one of the distinctive features of critical research is that the kinds of questions asked relate to the dynamics of power and exploitation in ways that potentially are linked to practical interventions and transformations'. Practice staff are employed by GPs, who may not see the immediate benefits of clinical supervision for their staff, particularly if it takes them away from their workplace. This is a typical example of how an action research project can be threatened by management and bureaucratic obstacles. The action researcher would therefore need to work with the advanced nurse practitioner as well as practice staff so that they could become sufficiently emancipated to negotiate the need for clinical supervision with general practitioners. The fact-finding stage would involve advanced practitioners and practitioners analysing the current position in relation to their clinical supervision needs; GPs might also be involved in this process to enable them to appreciate the value of clinical supervision. The group would then move through the action stages of planning, acting, observing and reflecting, while making necessary changes as they moved through the process.

Getting research into practice using critical research methods

The very essence of critical research ensures that research and practice are brought together. Involving participants in the research process in a way that is emancipatory results in changes being implemented *by* the people *for* the people. The researcher's task is to act as an advocate and to use the research process to effect change, rather than merely to describe the scene, as is typical in descriptive research, or to explore relationships between variables as is typical of exploratory research.

SUMMARY AND CONCLUSION

There are many ways of getting research into practice. This chapter focused on some approaches to research that demonstrate variations in proximity between the researcher and the research field. It would seem that the closer the researcher is to the field, the easier it is to bring about change and to get research into practice. Action research is an example of how the change process itself will cause change to take place. The different types of evaluation research illustrate how the distance between the researcher and the researched can vary. Goal-orientated approaches, such as those described in Chapter 11 using experiments, may require that 'getting research into practice' is a separate enterprise after the findings have been documented. A utility-orientated approach, however, involves all stakeholders and therefore there is less distance between the researcher and the field. Finally, use of critical research is an example of how research *exists* in practice through the experience of the participants. This chapter has illustrated how getting research into practice need not be an onerous task, but may be considered to be part of the research process itself.

REFERENCES

Adams C, Thomas E 2001 The benefits of integrated nursing teams in primary care. British Journal of Community Nursing 6(5): 271–274

Alvesson M, Sköldberg K 2001 Reflexive methodology: new vistas for qualitative research. Sage, London

Ashburner L, Birch K, Latimer J, Scrivens E 1997 Nurse practitioners in primary care. Centre for Health Planning and Management, Keele University, Keele

Baileff A 2000 Integrated nursing teams in primary care. Nursing Standard 14(48): 41–44

Balling K, McCubbin M 2001 Hospitalized children with chronic illness: parental care giving needs and valuing parental expertise. Journal of Paediatric Nursing: Nursing Care of Children and Families 16(2): 110–119

Bishop V 1997 Clinical supervision in practice. Macmillan, London

Bond M, Holland S 1998 Skills of clinical supervision for nurses. Open University Press, Buckingham

Boudieu P 1991 Language and symbolic power. Harvard University, Cambridge, MA

Burns R B 2000 Introduction to research methods. Sage, London

Butterworth T, Woods D 1999 Clinical governance and clinical supervision: working together to ensure safe and accountable practice: a briefing paper. School of Nursing Midwifery and Health Visiting, University of Manchester, Manchester

Clarke A, Dawson R 1999 Evaluation research: an introduction to principles, methods and practice. Sage, London

Daly W M, Carnwell R 2003 Nursing roles and levels of practice: a framework for differentiating between elementary, specialist and advancing nursing practice. Journal of Clinical Nursing 12: 158–167

Department of Health 1990 National Health Service and Community Care Act. HMSO, London

Department of Health 1993a New world new opportunities. HMSO, London

Department of Health 1993b A vision for the future: the nursing, midwifery and health visiting contribution to health and healthcare. HMSO, London

Department of Health 1997 The new NHS: modern dependable. HMSO, London

Department of Health 1998 Our healthier nation. HMSO, London

Department of Health 1999 Making a difference. HMSO, London

Department of Health 2000 Making a difference: integrated working in primary care. HMSO, London

Department of Health 2001 Primary care general practice and the NHS plan: information for GPs, nurses and other professionals and staff working in general practice in England. HMSO, London

Elcock K 1996 Consultant nurse: an appropriate title for the advanced nurse practitioner? British Journal of Healthcare 5(22): 1376

Faugier J, Butterworth C 1994 Position paper on clinical supervision. School of Nursing Studies, University of Manchester, Manchester

Forester J 1992 Critical ethnography: on fieldwork in a Habermasian way. In: Alversson M, Willmott H (eds) Critical management studies. Sage, London

Forrester S, Kline R 1997 Integrated nursing teams. Health Visitor 70(6): 229–231

Fowler J 1996 The organisation of clinical supervision within the nursing profession: a review of the literature. Journal of Advanced Nursing 32: 471–478

Frost S 1998 Perspectives on advanced practice: an educationalist's view. In: Rolfe G, Fulbrook P (eds) Advanced nursing practice. Butterworth-Heinemann, Oxford

Giddens A 1984 The constitution of society. University of California Press, Berkeley

Grundy S 1982 Three modes of action research. Curriculum Perspectives 2(3): 23–34

Guba E G, Lincoln Y S 1994 Competing paradigms in qualitative research. In: Denzin N K, Lincoln Y S (eds) Handbook of qualitative research. Sage, London

Hart E, Bond M 1995 Action research for health and social care: a guide to practice. Open University Press, Buckingham

Hicks C M 1990 Research and statistics: a practical introduction for nurses. Prentice-Hall, New York

Johns C 1993 Professional supervision. Journal of Nursing Management 1: 9–18

Kadushin A 1985 Supervision in social work. Columbia Press, New York

Kagan N, Werner A 1977 Supervision in psychiatric education. In: Kurpius D J, Baker R D, Thomas I D (eds) Supervision in applied training. Greenwood Press, London

Kilminster S M, Jolly B C 2000 Effective supervision in clinical practice settings: a literature review. Medical Education 34(10): 827–840

Kinnersley P, Anderson E, Parry K et al 2000 Randomised controlled trial of nurse practitioner versus general practitioner care for patients requesting 'same day' consultations in primary care. British Medical Journal 320(7241): 1043–1048

Kings Fund 1994 Seamless care or patchwork quilt? Discharging patients from acute hospital care. King's Fund Institute, London

Lewin K 1947a Frontiers in group dynamics I: concept method and reality in social science social equilibria and social change. Human Relations 1(1): 5–41

Lewin K 1947b Frontiers in group dynamics II: channels of group life social planning and action research. Human Relations 1(2): 143–153

Malin N A 2000 Evaluating clinical supervision in community homes and teams serving adults with learning disabilities. Journal of Advanced Nursing 313: 548–557

Marcus G 1986 Contemporary problems of ethnography in the modern world system. In: Guilford J, Marcus G (eds) Writing culture. University of California Press, Berkeley

Milne D, Oliver V 2000 Flexible formats of clinical supervision: description evaluation and implementation. Journal of Mental Health 93: 291–304

Mirr M 1995 Evaluating the effectiveness of advanced practice. In: Snyder M, Mirr P (eds) Advanced nursing practice: a guide to professional development. Springer, New York

Morrow R A 1994 Critical theory and methodology: contemporary social theory. Sage, London, vol. 3

Mundinger M O, Kane R L, Lenz E R et al 2000 Primary care outcomes in patients treated by nurse practitioners or physicians: a randomized trial. Journal of the American Medical Association 283(1): 59–68

NHSE 1997 Personal medical services: pilots under the NHS primary care act 1997: a comprehensive guide. Stationery Office, London

Nursing Midwifery Council (NMC) (2003) http://www.nmc.org.uk

Office of Technology Assessment 1986 Nurse practitioners physician's assistants and certified nurse-midwives: a policy analysis health technology care study. 37 OTA-HCS-37, US Government Printing Office, Washington DC

Olsen R, Maslin-Prothero P 2001 Dilemmas in the provision of own-home respite support for parents of young children with complex healthcare needs: evidence from an evaluation. Journal of Advanced Nursing 34(5): 603–610

Øvretveit J 2000 Evaluating health interventions. Open University Press, Buckingham

Owen J M, Rogers P J 1999 Programme evaluation: forms and approaches. Sage, London

Parlett M, Hamilton D 1976 Evaluation as illumination: a new approach to the study of innovatory programmes. In: Glass G V (ed) Evaluation Studies Review Annual, vol. 1. Sage, Beverly Hills

Patton M Q 1997 Utilisation-focused evaluation: the new century text. Sage, London

Perrow C 1978 Demystifying organizations. In: Sarri R, Heskenfield Y (eds) The management of human services. Columbia University Press, New York

Rink E, Ross F, Furne A 2000 Integrated nursing teams in primary care. Clinical Monograph no. 49. Nursing Times Books, London

Sartain S A, Maxwell M J, Todd P J, Haycox A R, Bundred P E 2001 Users' views on hospital and home care for acute illness in childhood. Health and Social Care in the Community 9(2): 108–117

Scriven M 1972 Pros and cons about goal-free evaluation. Evaluation Comment: The Journal of Educational Evaluation. Centre for Study of Evaluation, University of California, Los Angeles 34: 1–7

Snyder M, Mirr M (eds) 1995 Advancing healthcare practice. Springer, New York

Thomas J 1993 Doing critical ethnography. Sage, London

United Kingdom Central Council for Nursing, Midwifery and Health Visiting (UKCC) 1990 The report of the post-registration education and practice project. United Kingdom Central Council, London

United Kingdom Central Council for Nursing, Midwifery and Health Visiting 1994 The future of professional practice: the council's standards for education and practice following registration. United Kingdom Central Council, London

Veeramah R 2002 The benefits of using clinical supervision. Mental Health Nursing 22(1): 18–23

Venning P, Durie A, Roland M, Roberts C, Leese B 2000 Randomised controlled trial comparing cost effectiveness of general practitioners and nurse practitioners in primary care. British Medical Journal 320(7241): 1048–1053

Weaver M 2001 Introducing clinical supervision. British Journal of Podiatry 4(4): 134–143

Wilson-Barnett J, Barriball K L, Reynolds H, Jowett S, Ryrie I 2000 Recognising advancing nursing practice: evidence from two observational studies. International Journal of Nursing Studies 37(5): 389–400

FURTHER READING

Carnwell R 1997 Evaluation research. Churchill Livingstone, Edinburgh

PART 2

Practical experiences

PART CONTENTS

6

The physiotherapy experience

Pat Wrightson

Editors' comment

This chapter gives an overview of the developing research agenda in physiotherapy. Physiotherapy is one of the professions referred to in the UK as the allied health professions. This account demonstrates quite clearly the evolution of a profession, and tracks the development of education processes from the practice base of the NHS through to the present graduate-level education. It illustrates the importance of the interface between higher education and clinical areas in creating support networks that facilitate research developments in healthcare. The relatively recent history of research in the profession sets the scene for an account of the development of one academic unit of physiotherapy. This gives useful insights into some of the challenges faced by those working in academia who are given a remit to support research in practice.

INTRODUCTION

While some healthcare disciplines in the UK have a long association with higher education, many others have only relatively recently moved training and education programmes from a health service base to the university sector. In a text such as this it is important that consideration is given to such professional evolution, for, as indicated in Chapter 1, factors associated with increased uptake and utilization of research are closely linked to education preparation and support from experienced academic staff who can advise and support research activity. Consequently, education underpins the capacity of healthcare professions to develop and use research expertise.

The focus in this chapter is on one professional group, physiotherapy. Physiotherapy is the largest of 12 professions that make up a group collectively referred to as the 'allied health professions'. The profession's transition from a health service to a university based education programme in recent years encapsulates, in a relatively short time span, the experience of many healthcare professional groups. The challenges in research development faced by this group reflect those experienced by many other health professions, including nursing, and so can be usefully applied to diverse professional situations. In summary, this chapter gives a concise overview of the challenges faced in developing education and integrating research programmes with healthcare colleagues.

The first part of the chapter gives a brief historical perspective of the development of the physiotherapy profession and how this has influenced the professional drive to deliver evidence-based healthcare to meet the national research and development agenda (Peckham 1991) (see Ch. 2). To illustrate how this group has worked to foster research and development in one location, there is a case study of the strategic developments undertaken as one school of physiotherapy was relocated into a university school of health sciences (Department of Health 1989a).

HISTORY OF THE PROFESSION

The physiotherapy profession was founded in 1894 by four nurses fully trained in massage and medical rubbing (Wicksteed 1948). Since its modest beginnings, the profession has continued to grow in strength and importance, developing a range of skills and defining a body of knowledge, specifically in relation to musculoskeletal, neurological and respiratory care.

Until the 1990s physiotherapy education focused principally on training students to complete a curriculum of study and assessment defined by the Chartered Society of Physiotherapy (CSP) and the Council for Professions Supplementary to Medicine (CPSM). The title Chartered Society of Physiotherapy, which remains current, was adopted in 1942. With the founding of the National Health Service (NHS) in 1948, the CSP's training and examinations were approved as qualifications for employment within the NHS, and those who passed were known as chartered physiotherapists.

In the early years the medical profession had authority of control that extended to physiotherapists who, together with seven other occupational groups, were classed as medical auxiliaries. They included, for example, radiography, chiropody, occupational therapy. The medical profession's role with regard to direction, prescription, training and supervision at this time was considerable (Jones 1991). In due course the Professions Supplementary to Medicine Act of 1960 was passed, setting up the CPSM. The Physiotherapists' Board, one of eight constituent boards, assumed responsibility for inspection of schools of physiotherapy within the NHS, approving changes to the curriculum of study and assessment procedures which the CSP proposed. This represented a milestone in the physiotherapy profession's struggle towards professional autonomy.

Between 1960 and 1975 few major changes occurred, though a number of reports were commissioned which have influenced the development of the professions; for example closer integration of the education and practice of physiotherapy with occupational therapy and with the development of a degree course was proposed (CPSM 1970). The Tunbridge Report (Department of Health and Social Security 1972) disagreed, and emphasized the dominant role of the medical profession. The professions, however, refused to endorse this view. The Burt Report (CPSM 1973) endorsed the recommendations made by the CPSM in 1970 and, interestingly from the perspective of this chapter, also highlighted the need for the professions to conduct research into professional practice (CPSM 1973). The McMillan Report (Department of Health and Social Security 1973) endorsed the findings of the Burt Report, while also proposing self-management and clinical responsibility for these professions.

Following the Burt Report (CPSM 1973), physiotherapy has continued to develop both clinically and managerially with growing recognition of the role of chartered physiotherapists in clinical differential diagnosis, and instigation of progressive treatment programmes. Publication of a code of practice in 1977 confirmed the maturation of the profession by recognizing the rights of physiotherapists to make their own decisions on prescribing appropriate forms of physiotherapy for patients referred to them by medical practitioners, and also their right to terminate treatment (Department of Health and Social Security 1977). This significant change was further reinforced by publication in 1986 of a revised *Rules of Professional Conduct* (CSP 1986). Further revision in 1996 specified that physiotherapists should only practice in areas where they had appropriate education and experience to work safely and competently (CSP 1996). Another revision of the rules was published in 2002 (CSP 2002), the revisions reflecting the role and responsibilities of physiotherapists working within a wider framework of clinical governance (Department of Health 1998a).

In 1996, 36 years after the 1960 Professions Supplementary to Medicine Act, the National Health Service Executive (NHSE) commissioned a review of the operation of the statutory bodies established under the act. A further 5 years elapsed before a document was published, outlining the proposal for legislation to establish a new Health Professions Council (Department of Health 2001a). The review places protection of patients and the public at the centre of care and is part of a much wider government review for modernizing the regulation of health professions, with an aspiration to provide better healthcare (Department of Health 2001b). The Health Professions Council was formally established in 2002.

IMPACT OF HEALTH POLICY ON PHYSIOTHERAPY EDUCATION

Department of Health reforms of the late 1980s and early 1990s emphasized 'patient focused care' (Department of Health 1989a). A range of developments were noted including a shift to care in the community, with increased audit of patient progress, and identification of the need for outcome measures (Department of Health 1989b, 1989c, 1989d). A vision of 'integrated' care was further developed in the late 1990s (Department of Health 1997) and an improvement in health of the population was seen as a priority (Department of Health 1998a). Subsequent White Papers have set out an agenda for the 21st century that enables all members of the population to access quality care, delivered to defined and measurable standards (Department of Health 1998b). As indicated in Chapters 2 and 3, these developments were linked to an NHS research and development agenda with funding being allocated on the basis of priorities and needs in health service delivery (Department of Health 2000a).

Staff development is clearly linked to service development for, in order to achieve the healthcare objective, the *NHS Plan* (Department of Health 2000b) highlighted the need for planned investment and, critically, stressed the need for reform in the roles of professional staff. The clear message was that to achieve healthcare targets, new ways of working were required (Department of Health 2000b). The importance of physiotherapists in taking forward these agendas is evident from the strategy for allied health professionals set out in *Meeting the Challenge* (Department of Health 2000c). Physiotherapists will need to have the skills to deliver evidence-based healthcare (Department of Health 2000c). For the physiotherapy profession this highlighted the need to define a strategy to facilitate research into practice and provide evidence to support the efficacy of established practice. Educational changes had already begun and the time was now right to capitalize on the knowledge and skills developed in the new generations of physiotherapists.

Transition from diploma to degree

As a result of health and social reforms, changes to the NHS and changes in the higher education sector, there have been significant changes in the education and practice of physiotherapy (Potts 1996). In early years of physiotherapy practice professional qualification was an award of the CSP (i.e. a member of the CSP). In 1984 the CSP published guidelines signalling the move towards internal assessment of a graduate diploma in physiotherapy within NHS schools of physiotherapy, with a shift towards academic relocation evolving with the requirement that physiotherapy students should be educated to a level credited by the higher education sector as degree level (CSP 1984). This process was completed with the introduction of an all-graduate entry to the profession in 1992. This opened access to higher education and supported the development of an environment where students could be encouraged to develop independent learning skills and be responsible for their own learning, traits and characteristics of degree-level learning. Completion of a degree has ensured that all students are required to develop an understanding of critical appraisal skills including the ability to critique research literature. To support this learning, these insights are nurtured, aspects that are important if the physiotherapy profession is to take an active part in developing healthcare research.

Development of critical appraisal skills has been essential to the transformation from clinically based studies seeking technical competence in the 'traditional' physiotherapy programme to clinical practice based upon a sound knowledge base and clinical reasoning skills (Higgs 1992a). However, a mismatch between learning in academic and clinically based modules was a potential difficulty in the earlier years as the majority of clinical educators in physiotherapy had completed a diploma course, with few having completed a first degree (Cross 1992). Hence their understanding of research methodology, for example, would not reflect the student experience. While it is acknowledged that both students and clinical educators have a responsibility for managing learning in clinical modules (Higgs 1992b, 1993), the need to ensure reinforcement of learning from the context of critical appraisal of research was a particular challenge.

It would be necessary to develop learning strategies in degree programmes that would produce physiotherapists with good interpersonal skills, as well as the ability to enhance team-building, manage conflict and use information technology to support their work (McCoy 1991). These broader competencies are also essential to the development of an evidence-based culture in which clinical staff not only have to be able to access information but need to know what to do if new knowledge demands new approaches to care. This is where interpersonal skills, team working and conflict management interface with research activities (see Ch. 4).

Supporting learning

It is also important to note that the quality of learning of new graduates will be influenced by the capability of lecturers. Helping new students to understand research created a different challenge for lecturers, as staff who worked in NHS environments were not traditionally expected to develop expertise in research. For many former teachers of physiotherapy the need to upgrade their academic qualifications coincided with the implementation of a degree programme for new physiotherapy students. A survey of physiotherapy lecturers in England undertaken in 1994 gathered responses from 18 institutions. The survey confirmed that a high proportion of lecturing staff held or were undertaking a degree qualification, predominantly a taught masters degree. Only five institutions had one or two members of staff who held a PhD (Wrightson 1995). As with other aspects of the experience of transition, this was not just an issue for physiotherapy; the same issue had been identified in, for example, nursing (Clifford 1997).

This situation meant that strategic planning was necessary to ensure that students were not disadvantaged while lecturers' learning was being facilitated. Student support at the outset of graduate education in physiotherapy was addressed by teaching relating to research methods being enriched by university staff from different academic disciplines who had a background in research working alongside physiotherapy lecturers with higher degrees.

PHYSIOTHERAPY RESEARCH

As can be seen above, the total transition of physiotherapy education from health service to a higher education base can be tracked over a relatively short time period. This impacts upon the extent to which the profession has been able to contribute to healthcare research to date, as we see in the historical review below.

Historical perspective

Research in physiotherapy in the UK is relatively recent. Before 1975 there was little research into physiotherapy and published research relating to physiotherapy was led by medical practitioners (CSP 1992). This illustrated the need for physiotherapists to become involved in research (Rogers 1976, Metters 1978). As will be seen below, even by 1990 the health professional literature still showed only a few articles relating to physiotherapy.

A research interest group of physiotherapists was established in 1976 and worked to encourage the development of research into physiotherapy (CSP 1992). At about the same time the Department of Health recognized the lack of evidence-based practice and provided some early support in 1978 by setting up a limited number of Department of Health fellowships for members of the professions allied to medicine to undertake research training (CSP 1992). This was followed in 1983 by the setting up of the Centre for Physiotherapy Research based at King's College, London. The Department of Health and Social Security provided funding to the centre to carry out applied research into physiotherapy practice (CSP 1992).

Research developments in the main have been driven by the educational sector, where research is an integral part of academic activity. Clinical research had been much more limited and the early posts for research physiotherapists were generally in collaboration with medical research projects. Equally, physiotherapists wishing to develop their research skills by completing doctoral studies had in many instances completed their studies in academic departments whose areas of research expertise were related to physiotherapy, such as physiology, psychology or medicine. Due to the relative recency of physiotherapy departments in universities, many physiotherapists involved in postdoctoral research have done their research in associated academic areas, potentially removing them from easy access by clinical physiotherapists wishing to undertake research. Overall, however, it is interesting to note that the research skill mix of physiotherapy staff changed very rapidly. By 1996, over 40 chartered physiotherapists held a

PhD, and these included both university lecturers and clinical physiotherapists (Potts 1996); a total of 102 were identified in 2001 (Illott & Bury 2002).

CSP research strategy

In order to promote and develop physiotherapy research and support physiotherapists undertaking research, the CSP published a research strategy (CSP 1995). The policy statement recognized that physiotherapy is a service provided within a competitive market and one in which cost-effectiveness is an important issue. Therefore, research is needed to provide evidence of the effectiveness of physiotherapy and the health benefits to clients. A reassuring feature of this statement for many physiotherapists was the recognition that not every physiotherapist would be involved in undertaking original research. Emphasis was placed on all physiotherapists having research awareness and being able to access and implement information from other people's research activity. The strategy also promoted the importance of a wide range of relevant activity, recognizing that research could be both 'pure' and 'applied' (see Chs 1 and 2).

For research to grow it needed to develop in collaboration with established researchers from health and social backgrounds and be directed towards the priorities of the NHS research and development strategy, at both national and local levels (Peckham 1991). For many, the initial route has been to develop research related to the local NHS research and development agendas, which have been valuable in promoting understanding of local healthcare issues, and thus more likely to attract funding. Difficulties for the allied health professions are the small size of the individual professions when compared to, for example, nursing, and their lack of representation on key decision-making bodies. For example, allied health professions were rarely represented on research directorates within the NHS although this is now being rectified in some NHS clinical units and the increase in multiprofessional approaches to research (see Chs 1 and 12) is seen as a positive step.

The CSP research strategy highlighted the need for research awareness and practice in the clinical setting. Collaboration between university lecturers and clinical physiotherapists has been essential to developing clinically based research to underpin practice. The strategy paper concluded by identifying 14 priorities, which addressed activities needed to develop research within undergraduate and postgraduate education, recognizing that it was part of continuing professional development. These included: activity to secure increased funding for physiotherapy research; developing the society's information resource centre; developing links with the NHS Centre for Reviews and Dissemination, the Cochrane Collaboration Centre and the Projects Register System, and a review and improvement of its journal and fact sheets to promote dissemination of information (see Ch. 4). All of these have been achieved in the ensuing years. Recent publication of *Priorities for Physiotherapy Research in the UK* confirms the profession's desire to increase research activity.

Recognizing the value of interdisciplinary research and the value of critical mass, the CSP has joined with other non-medical health professions that have been collectively renamed allied health professions (AHPs) (Department of Health 2000c) to publish a research strategy. The Allied Health Professions Forum has proposed a national coordinated system for improving the research capacity and productivity of the AHPs. The CSP states: 'This is a landmark document in the history of research and development for the Allied Health Professions' (CSP 2001, p. 1).

Approaches to research in physiotherapy

A range of research methods can be identified in published reports of research activity examining physiotherapy practice. These give the profession a source for lively debate and, as professional confidence has increased over the last decade, the topic of which research methodologies are most appropriate has challenged many (Parry 1991). Early research tended to follow the example of well-established research groups in healthcare, for example medicine and psychology, applying the principles of experimental research to physiotherapy practice as a means of developing the knowledge base of physiotherapy. However, with increasing insight into the diverse aspects of practice, many physiotherapists, alongside other health professionals, believe that a qualitative approach may be more appropriate in certain care situations (Shepard 1992).

Other approaches have come under review. For example, an evolving interest which has developed from research in psychology is the use of a single case study approach, to identify whether a single individual is benefiting from treatment. A series of similar case studies provides more detailed evidence of the efficacy of an intervention (Barlow & Hersen 1984, Riddoch 1991). While debates as to the relative merits of varied approaches continue, as professional confidence in research has grown so has the recognition that the most appropriate approach will be determined by the research question asked. The need for physiotherapists to develop skills in varied approaches is essential to ensure that research is developed in a way that is relevant to physiotherapy practice. Physiotherapy research needs to inform and support the philosophy of current healthcare delivery. Richardson (1995, p. 544) supports the view that both qualitative and quantitative research are necessary to 'acknowledge both the technical judgment and the interpersonal management of treatment and to develop both the science and art of physiotherapy practice. More studies based within an interpretive paradigm would balance the professional profile of research and help to assure the quality of the physiotherapy service and effectiveness of its delivery'.

Growth in professional knowledge and expertise has also led to the recognition that research is not an isolated activity, but is undertaken most successfully in teams where a breadth of complementary research skills can be applied to determine the most relevant methodology. This factor is well recognized now in the increased development of interprofessional working in research, an approach supported by many funding bodies (see Chs 1, 2 and 12).

Parry (1997) stressed that research must address the needs of individual clients, and also suggested that individual physiotherapists were likely to base their research questions on their own experiences, including the particular type of research methodology. The need to provide quality care to all patients, based upon the best evidence (Department of Health 1998a), has given impetus for research to promote evidence-based healthcare and clinical effectiveness. Evidence-based healthcare involves researchers and practitioners, but to be successful must also include policy makers and users (Bury & Mead 1998).

Research in clinical practice

Healthcare has continued to develop from the 1989 NHS reforms. The publication of the White Paper *The New NHS* (Department of Health 1997) continued the development of primary care. The Green Paper *Our Healthier Nation* (Department of Health 1998b) set out proposals to improve people's living conditions and health, while recognizing that individuals also have a responsibility to contribute to their own well-being. The philosophy of healthcare has made a major shift towards quality care (Department of Health 1998a), which is patient-focused care (Department of Health 2000b), promoting health (Department of Health 1998b), creating patient autonomy and empowering patients in self-care.

Development of research activity within clinical practice is essential to give credibility to many aspects of physiotherapy. Also the ethos of the NHS has meant that managers need to investigate, set and maintain standards (Department of Health 1998a) to provide a cost-effective and efficient service which is responsive to local needs. Those seeking to commission health services want to know more about the value of the service provided. Within this environment staff are required critically to appraise their work, objectively analyse outcome measures and be part of a system of professional audit which supports clinical practice. This provides a challenge for all healthcare workers, including physiotherapists, as not all staff wish to be involved in these activities which are often seen as closely akin to research. However, all staff today do need to have a basic understanding of research methods to help them in critically appraising their work in the light of existing published research which contributes to the development of the knowledge base of practice.

Linking clinical practice, research and education

Before the 1990s, physiotherapists qualified following a period of training and were not generally exposed to research and research methods. Research opportunities were limited, and many physiotherapists required advice and support to enable them to undertake research activity. Officers of the CSP initially played an active role in promoting more widely members' understanding of evidence-based practice by holding a series of workshops promoting clinical effectiveness throughout Britain (Mead 1996). The aim was to provide the participants with an understanding of terminology, while guiding them through finding evidence on which practice could be based. The need to critically appraise research and other evidence to determine its reliability, prior to developing clinical guidelines, was a key aim of the workshops. Dissemination, implementation and evaluation were also covered as this is the means by which good research evidence is applied to practice (Mead 1996). As a result of these workshops clinical interest groups have developed evidence-based clinical guidelines. This is in line with the publication by the NHSE in 1996 of the document *Using Clinical Guidelines*. Professional bodies are expected to develop, maintain and endorse guidelines relating to practice. Dissemination of information on evidence-based practice in physiotherapy has continued to be promoted by the CSP's Current Awareness Bulletins and in recent times via the CSP website.

Richardson (1993) has attempted to clarify the links between education, practice and research in physiotherapy. It is suggested that as a profession we need to develop an exclusive theoretical basis for physiotherapy which can underpin and extend the limits of practice. From this perspective education is seen as a means of giving the capability to practice, whereas practice forms the basis of clinical research.

Research for Health (Department of Health 1993) summarized the progress made in 2 years. It highlighted the continuing need for problem-led research and the benefits of multidisciplinary research activities. Parry (1993) saw this as an opportunity not to be missed. She argued that for too long the profession had played 'second fiddle' to the medical and nursing professions; now there was an opportunity to collaborate in research activities which reflected physiotherapists' areas of interest. Thus the next stage in developing physiotherapy research was to encourage development in the widest sense. This challenged the interface between clinical practice and higher education.

Publications as a measure of research output

Some development of research was seen during the 1980s, with the number of publications increasing by the early 1990s (Richardson 1995). This can be linked to the redirection of the journal *Physiotherapy*, which seeks to advance physiotherapy through peer reviewed articles. By the 21st century the journal aimed to advance physiotherapy through publication of original research, critical reviews and scholarly papers, an aim which has been achieved (CSP 2003). The increased demand to disseminate research findings through published work by the allied health professions has supported the introduction of a number of new journals related to therapy and rehabilitation, for example *Physiotherapy Theory and Practice*, the *International Journal of Therapy and Research*, and the *Journal of Inter-professional Care*. These have provided another outlet for physiotherapists wishing to publish.

As a relatively new profession, the need for physiotherapy to explore its foundations and push forward its knowledge base are important. For this reason interpretative articles are increasingly welcomed in publication media. This relates to the skills of critical appraisal, as interpretation of research is an area for review and debate. There is a need for the profession to ensure that these skills are widely developed so that research information can be judged on a sound methodological basis (Shortfall 2002). As skills develop so the capacity for physiotherapists to ensure their practices are based on clear evidence increases and such development is increasingly apparent in practice today (Wiles 2003).

DEVELOPING THE ACADEMIC ENVIRONMENT

As discussed above, the key aspect of developing research in physiotherapy was to facilitate the academic preparation of the next generations of practitioners by the transition from diploma level preparation to degree level. Beyond this was the need to consider ways of increasing insights into research and practice through higher level study to masters degree and doctorate level. This sounds a relatively straightforward task, but it involved the need for much more diverse planning and consideration, as will be seen below. The following account seeks to illustrate this by drawing upon one experience in which an academic department of physiotherapy was created in a university in 1995. Shortly after the move to the university, the department of physiotherapy joined the existing department of nursing to form a school of health sciences.

Developing the strategy

How was the school to move forward, what were its strengths and weaknesses? What opportunities and threats existed? Key issues were considered at a school 'away day', from which a framework for a research and development strategy developed. This was published in 1998. A number of targets were identified, many of which highlighted the importance of the 'development' part of the strategy for physiotherapy lecturers. A culture of research needed to be fostered in which an increase in the ratio of staff described as 'research active' was essential (in university settings 'research active' means that staff are involved in developing and reporting on research projects). It was necessary too to consider preparation of staff to doctoral level and beyond. Research publications were also reviewed as these are the external measure of research output, and it was proposed that the number of these in peer reviewed academic journals should be increased (see Chs 1 and 12).

Ability to support students undertaking higher degrees by research was another goal that had to be met. The importance of integrating research activity undertaken by undergraduate and postgraduate students into the school's research agenda was viewed as concurrent activity. Identification of research themes, developing collaborative links with other schools both within the university and externally, and increasing the number of peer reviewed grants awarded to the school were viewed as activity consistent with the appointment to a lecturing post. Goals deemed to be longer term were to increase the number of peer reviewed grants awarded to staff, to increase the number of students registered to undertake research degrees, and to establish quality assurance mechanisms to monitor the quality of research and development activity in the school (School of Health Sciences 1998).

Staffing issues

From the perspective of research developments, the need to contribute to the development of the 'body of knowledge' for physiotherapy was clear at the outset. This reflects the academic mission of many 'research-led' universities, that is those universities that generate large volumes of research to a level that is considered to be of national or international standard (HEFCE 2001a). Consequently, there was a need to explore ways in which the relocation of physiotherapy from a health service to a higher education setting could support the development of research expertise. It was important to consider this from the perspective of staff development, education and, managerially, exploring ways in which research developments would be funded and managed.

From another perspective it was also important to find ways of working with NHS colleagues to develop the research agenda for physiotherapy. Linked with this was a need to explore ways of working collaboratively with colleagues in the multidisciplinary healthcare team to meet new ideologies in research (see Chs 1 and 12). The location of physiotherapy alongside nursing, a profession that has been identified as facing similar challenges in developing research (Department of Health 2001b), was helpful as it facilitated a pooling of resources and expertise for mutual benefit and leadership from which research and development has been implemented.

Education developments

There was a need to think beyond degree level and consider how broader academic developments would be facilitated. It was noted that if students were to be educated to degree level it would also be important to support the education of the clinical practitioners who might be supporting them to at least degree, and preferably to masters, level of study. If such opportunities were to be created for this group then the development of a new lecturer workforce was an essential prerequisite to developing the academic agenda from the university setting.

As the move to the university sector had been anticipated for some time there had been an opportunity to ensure that teaching staff were appropriately prepared for new roles in which university lecturing contracts specified research, teaching and administrative duties. All staff had relevant professional and teaching qualifications, with five holding a first degree, seven a masters degree, three in the process of completing masters level studies, and two registered for a PhD (Wrightson 1996). This was a good starting point from which to develop strategies for the further academic development of physiotherapy. The opportunity was there to develop a strategy that addressed staffing and research training at undergraduate and postgraduate level.

Research development for academic staff

In transferring a group of teaching staff from roles involving teaching in the NHS to lecturing roles in a university it was important to foster understanding that the roles of university lecturers are more diverse. Research was a new dimension of this work for many staff. It was anticipated that not all staff who transferred from the NHS would wish to be classed as researchers because this did not reflect aspects of their career development to date in their NHS roles. However, it was essential that the close relationship between teaching and research was acknowledged (see Ch. 1). Knowledge is developed through research giving teachers the professional insights they require to facilitate learning in their students. The aim was to develop a culture of scholarship in the school that acknowledged the diverse backgrounds of lecturing staff. Moreover, in addition to the challenge of taking a proactive role in contributing to the knowledge developed through research, there was the need to focus on ways in which existing knowledge in teaching and practice in physiotherapy could be analyzed and used. At this time there was a strong push to address the evidence-based agenda in healthcare and one of the PhD qualified physiotherapists was allocated to join regional development initiatives to support physiotherapy research activity (see Ch. 2).

The processes involved in staff development to support research are ongoing and will remain a key feature of the school research strategy for many years to come. This need can be tracked to the recent history of the profession, outlined above, which demonstrates that a number of academic healthcare departments have some 'catching up' to do in this field (Department of Health 2001b).

Development involves ensuring that academic staff have a first foot on the ladder and are able to access the necessary training to develop their knowledge and skill in research. Consequently the revised school research strategy (School of Health Sciences 2001) involves ensuring that support is provided for staff to undertake masters and doctoral studies. This is an ongoing process as new staff are constantly joining the team. However, this strategy has helped ensure that all staff hold a higher degree and several members of staff now have PhDs, with an increasing number having started this process. It is recognized that in the majority of schools within the university a much greater proportion of academic staff hold doctoral qualifications and it is anticipated that in due course this profile will be reflected in physiotherapy. However, as preparation at this level is a long and often slow process, realistic goals must be set. Simply by referring back to the modern history of the physiotherapy profession it is possible to see that it would be unrealistic to set staff skill mix targets, in terms of research development, that were commensurate, for example, with schools such as psychology or physiology, since these disciplines have a much longer history of academic development within the higher education sector.

Staff development activities are supported by a programme of staff development review interviews. These enable staff to discuss ways of balancing their professional aspirations to undertake formal study, such as those for doctoral qualifications, with ideas they may have to develop research objectives that are measurable and achievable. Critical to this process is the need to demonstrate research output through publishing research activity. A number of staff have elected to concentrate on teaching and administrative roles, transferring to a lecturer contract that specifies 'teaching only', although scholarship is recognized as an important aspect of this role. However, for younger members of academic staff, there is perhaps greater pressure to complete doctoral studies.

Another strategy that was developed early in this process was making available a 3-month period of study leave, to assist with the writing up stage of research. Again this has yielded positive outcomes, enabling staff to complete their research reports sooner than might otherwise be possible.

Following completion of a PhD, a research student would normally undertake a postdoctoral post within a supportive research environment, focusing on their area of research. Current under-funding of nursing and physiotherapy research means that this is not possible (HEFCE 2001b). The challenge of finding funds to support postdoctoral studies in healthcare professions remains, but encouragingly, on a national level, there is evidence of such funding being made available to physiotherapy research in a steadily incremental way. This is another strand of the local strategic development in which some success has been identified, with a variety of funding mechanisms enabling staff newly qualified at doctoral level to undertake research work.

In summary, at this local level, the profile of physiotherapy academic staff has changed from, in the 1980s, a largely diploma qualified staff to the current one where all staff have higher degrees at masters level and there is a steady increase of staff with doctorates. It will be some time before ratios match other disciplines in higher education where a 100% doctoral qualified staff may be the norm, but nonetheless, the fact that the profile has changed so much in a relatively short period of time is external evidence of the rapidly changing face of physiotherapy when viewed from the perspective of research knowledge.

The recent large increases in student commissions arising out of the *NHS Plan* (Department of Health 2000b) mean that all academic departments are required to increase their teaching capacity to support the educational needs of new physiotherapy students. While the challenges of meeting these educational needs should not be underestimated, the changes bring further opportunity to recruit staff at differing levels, from postgraduate research and teaching fellows through all grades to professor. The need to achieve a more diverse skill mix and profile of grades is important in establishing a dynamic team and, as teaching and research are now well integrated, this brings parallel opportunities to undertake further research developments.

Skill development

The ability to write, cost and submit research proposals is a skill that active researchers must develop. The majority of staff have completed part-time doctoral studies, in most cases working in relative isolation. They have therefore not been exposed to the process of researching and writing research bids that forms part of the business of working as one of an established research team. Development of staff ability has been through working on proposals with established researchers within this and other schools. The setting up of a number of small research awards in the school to support pilot work has required applicants to submit a detailed proposal for peer review; if applicants are successful, annual progress reports are required, with a detailed report on completion.

Other practical developments in the school include the introduction of different ways of disseminating research activity. This has enabled staff to share both the trials and tribulations of working on research projects and some of the practical aspects of trying to develop research expertise alongside teaching and administrative work. This is further supported by a steady increase in publications and conference presentations, and publishing in targeted journals. Here peer support networks have helped staff new to this process.

Research training at undergraduate and postgraduate levels

To foster and support physiotherapy research for the future, undergraduate and postgraduate students need to study a variety of research methodologies that equip them to undertake evidence-based practice. A review of the research methods modules within the school was undertaken, to provide an educational framework which demonstrated progression from undergraduate level 1, 2 and 3, through to level M for postgraduate students.

A research route on the masters programme opened up the opportunity for students to study research as a separate topic. Moreover, it meant that those registered to undertake higher research degrees (e.g. MPhil or PhD) had ready access to more formal programmes of study if required in addition to traditional supervisory support. Postgraduate study is currently being reviewed in the light of doctoral level D, with the development of a taught clinical doctorate programme (Quality Assurance Agency 2001). It is anticipated that such programmes will help with the development required for new posts such as consultant therapist posts. Byrne (2001) highlights the need for clinical staff to achieve a high level of research capability to underpin clinical practice.

The small number of physiotherapists who have completed the school's taught masters degree programme has meant that few publications of direct relevance to physiotherapy have been published at the time of writing, but the signs are that increasing demand and utilization of these programmes of study are beginning to reap rewards.

Today's students will be tomorrow's researchers, and it is imperative that research training of the highest standard is provided to meet the prevailing healthcare philosophies. In a world in which the focus is on client needs rather than role demarcation created by traditional practice (Department of Health 2000b) it is essential that practitioners learn to work together from an early stage in their career. The importance of multiprofessional research is now evident (CSP 2001) and to address this the continued review of research training in the school resulted in the introduction, in 2001, of shared research modules for undergraduate nursing and physiotherapy students. Opportunity to do this via research modules will hopefully reap rewards in terms of preparing this generation of students to think more widely and more creatively in generating research ideas, to use research in their practice and, for the few, to lead the research agenda in a proactive way.

WORKING WITH THE NHS

Another critical aspect of the school's research strategy was to find ways of working collaboratively with the NHS. The school actively sought to develop collaborative links with local NHS trusts, which were required to develop their nursing and therapy research activity, linked to NHS research and development priorities (see Ch. 2).

External support

Within the West Midlands, as part of the strategy to implement the NHS research and development agenda, a regional clinical trials unit was developed and staff were located in two research-led universities (see Ch. 2). Part funding for one of five senior research fellow posts was preferentially allocated to physiotherapy, an important post in acknowledging the needs of the group. The need for pump-priming to support development of clinically based research for this profession was considered essential.

The remit of the post was to provide support to all regional clinical trials in physiotherapy. Support available from this unit for clinical trials has been invaluable, consisting at the minimum of statistical support and database development, data inputting, report writing and the opportunity to access researchers experienced in clinical trials. Two physiotherapy clinical trials set up in conjunction with two local NHS trusts have resulted in the principal investigator undertaking a jointly funded lecturer/practitioner post based within the school of health sciences. Academic members of staff providing research support to these trials have gained personal development in clinical trials methodology through their involvement with the clinical trials unit.

Local action

A key action item arising from the school's 1998 research strategy was to develop collaborative links to support the research agenda with NHS trusts within the West Midlands. These links have been facilitated in a number of ways, for example honorary appointments to the school of key clinical staff were made. Within some of the larger trusts appointments have been made to research posts, and although the post holders have to date had a professional background in nursing, their remit is to promote nursing and therapy research. Their appointment to honorary posts within the school has provided the opportunity for a larger number of research-active staff to work collaboratively to support the NHS research agenda. Secondment of staff into the school on both a part-time and full-time basis has increased the number of successfully funded research bids. More recently, honorary appointments for two doctorally qualified staff to research units in local trusts is fostering increased collaboration in clinical research activity.

In order to promote research developments in physiotherapy and nursing, a number of research studies have been undertaken by the school within local NHS trusts which have identified the clinical staff needs in research. These have been followed by multiprofessional workshops related to developing research awareness and evidence-based practice. The workshops have provided an opportunity for a greater number of staff to develop their research awareness, while a number of physiotherapists continue to access formal research methods modules as part of a masters degree.

SUMMARY AND CONCLUSION

This chapter has explored the evolution of one professional group both professionally and specifically in the context of research. An account of the progress of one academic department has demonstrated some aspects of research development that have impacted upon research development in one locality. The inter-relationship of research with education and practice is important. From the perspective of physiotherapy, parallel developments in education and practice may prove to be beneficial in that they have promoted a shared responsibility for research development to underpin practice in clinical settings.

Developing physiotherapy research activity is a tremendous challenge for all concerned. The history and work reported here is only the first step in what may prove to be a major development in healthcare research. Physiotherapists face the same challenges as other members of the healthcare team in developing a sound evidence-base for future practice. However, as can be seen here, much has been achieved in a few short years and no doubt much more will be achieved in the years ahead.

REFERENCES

Barlow D H, Hersen M 1984 Single case experimental designs: strategies for studying behaviour change, 2nd edn. Pergamon Press, Oxford
Bury T, Mead J 1998 Evidence-based health care: a practical guide for therapists. Butterworth-Heinemann, Oxford
Byrne P 2001 One small step for physio, one giant leap for physiotherapy. Physiotherapy Frontline 8(6): 6
Chartered Society of Physiotherapy 1984 Guidelines for the approval of courses leading to the eligibility for membership of the Chartered Society of Physiotherapy. Chartered Society of Physiotherapy, London
Chartered Society of Physiotherapy 1986 Rules of professional conduct. Physiotherapy. Chartered Society of Physiotherapy, London
Chartered Society of Physiotherapy 1992 Policy statement. Physiotherapy research. Physiotherapy 78(5): 356–357
Chartered Society of Physiotherapy 1995 CSP research strategy. Policy statement. Physiotherapy 81(5): 285–289
Chartered Society of Physiotherapy 1996 Rules of professional conduct. CSP Professional Affairs Department, London
Chartered Society of Physiotherapy 2001 Allied health professions strategy. http://www.csp.org.uk/effectivepractice/research/publications [accessed 8 April 2003]
Chartered Society of Physiotherapy 2002 Rules of professional conduct, 2nd edn. Chartered Society of Physiotherapy/Lansdowne Press, London
Chartered Society of Physiotherapy 2003 The journal of the Chartered Society of Physiotherapy. Physiotherapy 89(3): 138–199
Clifford C 1997 Nurse teachers and research. Nurse Education Today 17(2): 115–120

Council for Professions Supplementary to Medicine 1970 Report and recommendations of the Remedial Professions Committee [Oddie Report]. Richard Madley, London

Council for Professions Supplementary to Medicine 1973 Report of the Remedial Professions Committee [Burt Report]. Richard Madley, London

Cross V 1992 Clinicians needs in clinical education: a report on a needs analysis workshop. Physiotherapy 78(10): 758–761

Department of Health 1989a Working for patients. Working Paper 2. Funding and contracts for hospital services. HMSO, London

Department of Health 1989b Working for patients. Working Paper 6. Medical audit. HMSO, London

Department of Health 1989c Working for patients. Working Paper 11. Framework for information systems overview. HMSO, London

Department of Health 1989d Caring for people. Community care in the next decade and beyond. HMSO, London

Department of Health 1993 Research for health. Department of Health, London

Department of Health 1997 The new NHS. Department of Health Publications, Wetherby, West Yorkshire

Department of Health 1998a A first class service: quality in the NHS. Department of Health, London

Department of Health 1998b Our healthier nation. A contract for health. Stationery Office, London

Department of Health 2000a Research and development for a first class service. NHS Research and Development Funding Branch, Department of Health, London

Department of Health 2000b The NHS plan: a plan for investment: a plan for reform. http://www.nhs.uk/nationalplan [accessed 11 August 2000]

Department of Health 2000c Meeting the challenge: a strategy for allied health professions. Department of Health Publications, London

Department of Health 2001a Establishing the new Health Professions Council. Department of Health, London

Department of Health 2001b Modernising regulation in the health professions. Department of Health Publications, London

Department of Health and Social Security 1972 Statement by the Committee on Remedial Professions [Tunbridge Report]. HMSO, London

Department of Health and Social Security 1973 The remedial professions: a report by a working party set up in March 1973 by the secretary for social services [McMillan Report]. HMSO, London

Department of Health and Social Security 1977 Health services development. Relationship between the medical and remedial professions. Health Circular (77): 33

Higgs J 1992a Developing clinical reasoning. Physiotherapy 78(8): 575–578

Higgs J 1992b Managing clinical education. The educator-manager and the self-directed learner. Physiotherapy 78(11): 822–828

Higgs J 1993 Managing clinical education: the programme. Physiotherapy 79(4): 239–246

Higher Education Funding Council for England 2001a A guide to the 2001 research assessment exercise. http://hero.ac.uk/rae/pubs/index.htm [accessed 10 February 2003]

Higher Education Funding Council for England 2001b Research in nursing and allied health professions: report of task group 3. HEFCE and Department of Health, London

Illott I, Bury T 2002 Research capacity: a challenge for the therapy professions. Physiotherapy 88(4): 194–200

Jones R J 1991 The growth of autonomy in physiotherapy. In: Jones R J (ed) Management in physiotherapy. Radcliffe Medical Press, Oxford, ch. 3, p. 18

McCoy 1991 A curriculum for the future. Physiotherapy 77(3): 181–182

Mead J 1996 Evidence based practice – how far have we come? Physiotherapy 82(12): 653–654

Metters J S 1978 Research in physiotherapy: the way forward. Physiotherapy 64(12): 364–367

National Health Service Executive 1996 Using clinical guidelines to improve patient care within the NHS. Department of Health, London

Parry A 1991 Physiotherapy and methods of inquiry: conflict and reconciliation. Physiotherapy 77(7): 435–438

Parry A 1993 The future is now: an opportunity or a threat. Physiotherapy 79(11): 753–754

Parry A 1997 New paradigms for old: musings on the shape of clouds. Physiotherapy 83(8): 423–433

Peckham M 1991 Research and development for the NHS. Lancet 338: 367–371

Potts J 1996 Physiotherapy in the next century: opportunities and challenges. Physiotherapy 82(3): 150–155

Quality Assurance Agency for Higher Education 2001 The framework for higher education qualifications in England, Wales and Northern Ireland. http://www.qaa.ac.uk/

Richardson B 1993 Practice, research and education – what is the link? Physiotherapy 79(5): 317–322

Richardson B 1995 Qualitative approaches to evaluating quality of service. Physiotherapy 81(9): 541–545

Riddoch J 1991 Evaluation and practice. Physiotherapy 77(7): 439–443

Rogers S 1976 A role for physiotherapists in research. Physiotherapy 62(4): 127–128

School of Health Sciences 1998 School of Health Sciences research strategy. School of Health Sciences, University of Birmingham, Birmingham, UK

School of Health Sciences 2001 School of Health Sciences research strategy. School of Health Sciences, University of Birmingham, Birmingham, UK

Shepard K F 1992 Alternative approaches to research in physical therapy: positivism and phenomenology. Physical Therapy 73(2): 88–97

Shortfall R 2002 Physiotherapists must improve their research appraisal skills [letter to the editor]. Physiotherapy 88(1): 64

Wicksteed J H 1948 The growth of a profession, being the history of the Chartered Society of Physiotherapy, 1894–1945. Edward Arnold, London, pp. 9–41

Wiles R 2003 Physiotherapy research foundation. Physiotherapy 89(3): 138–139

Wrightson P A 1996 The effects of NHS reforms on physiotherapy education and clinical practice. Unpublished Master of Social Science thesis, University of Birmingham, Birmingham, UK

7

The midwifery experience

Christine Henderson

Editors' comment

This chapter offers a comprehensive account of the challenges of developing a research agenda in the midwifery profession. A clear historical perspective is presented and the reader can trace the pattern of development as the profession moves from a position of minimal research towards evidence-based practice. The chapter is complemented by the presentation of an account that identifies the action taken by one women's healthcare trust to change the culture of their organization to become more evidence based. The account provides useful insights into the strategy employed.

INTRODUCTION

The principle of clinical effectiveness is a laudable aim that we are all striving for and yet it is one that is not easy to implement. There are many reasons for this, to do with the organization we work in, the influence and power of people within it and their perceptions of effective and appropriate care. Those using the services are being given more opportunities to become involved in how care is delivered. They have access to, and are being presented with, information about what is clinically effective, based on evidence. Indeed there are now specific courses for users of maternity services to develop critical appraisal skills in order to evaluate the reliability and validity of the available evidence about effective care (CCIT 1996). Sackett et al (1997) defined evidence-based practice as follows: 'Evidence Based Practice is the conscientious, explicit and judicious use of current best evidence in making decisions about the care of individual patients. The practice of evidence based healthcare means integrating individual clinical expertise with the best available external, clinical evidence from systematic research'. Without research evidence we risk being out of date in clinical practice and may jeopardize the quality of care that we give. Of course for many of the things we do the evidence may be inadequate or just not available. However, our judgements should be based on the best possible evidence available. This may include available research, opinion and/or our own experiences. Evidence-based practice is the 'in phrase' today and although there are sceptics who think it is a passing fashion there is every indication that the government means business. Healthcare must be founded upon the best possible evidence and therefore the Department of Health is investing large sums of money in research and development (R&D).

The purpose of this chapter is to:

- Review developments related to research in a midwifery context over the last 30 years
- Briefly look at issues to do with research in the midwifery programme with examples from five institutions
- Describe how a women's healthcare NHS trust is working towards adopting a research culture in its drive for clinical effectiveness.

BACKGROUND

It was the Briggs Report (Department of Health and Social Security 1972) that used the term 'research-based practice' which became part of the language of nurses, midwives and health visitors. The issues revolved around the education of nurses in research methods, developing critical thinking skills, increasing the output of studies and getting research into practice. In 1996 Hunt, in an editorial entitled 'Barriers to research utilisation' (Hunt 1996), referred to the same 'new' concept, now coming around again for the fourth or fifth time, that is the need for clinical practice to be research based. She highlighted the efforts in nursing over the previous 30 years to realize this. Although some of these developments had an incidental impact on midwifery, there were others more specific to midwifery worthy of note.

RESEARCH DEVELOPMENTS: A MIDWIFERY CONTEXT (1970s)

Research conducted prior to the 1970s was minimal and concerned the role, retention and recruitment of midwives, necessary because of staff shortages. The need for midwifery, alongside nursing, to become a research-based profession focused on the future preparation of the nursing professions, their education beyond registration and the regulation of nursing, midwifery and health visiting. Teachers with little knowledge or experience in this area were expected to teach students how to research, which led to research being an educator's nightmare. Some students and clinical midwives felt that this was a topic that might interest others but which was not for them (see Ch. 6).

In the wake of the Brigg's Report there followed a number of initiatives to take the question of research-based practice forward. Table 7.1 (pp. 132–133) summarizes events, developments and the focus of activities relevant to midwifery. Among these were the setting up of a number of research units for nursing some of which also had a focus in midwifery. Of great importance to midwifery was the establishment of the National Epidemiological Perinatal Unit (NEPU) at Oxford consisting of a multidisciplinary group who began compiling a register of controlled trials in perinatal medicine, which led to a systematic review of the evidence of effective care in pregnancy and childbirth. In addition, research studentships were introduced by the Department of Health and Social Security (DHSS) (see Ch. 2) and the Scottish Home and Health Department (SHHD), and a variety of scholarships were established, some specific to midwifery such as the Maws Educational Award and that offered by the Iolanthe Trust.

Research activity undertaken by midwives began to increase towards the end of the 1970s, although it should be noted that many studies were only small-scale and most were conducted as part of undergraduate and postgraduate studies rather than higher degrees in research or independent research activity. However, with this growth in research activity the need for dissemination of the findings of research studies assumed greater importance. Conferences focusing on research and the midwife in the UK were established in 1978 and were an important development in raising research awareness in the midwifery profession (Thomson & Robinson 1985).

THE 1980s: KNOWLEDGE AND APPRECIATION OF RESEARCH

The emphasis on educational appreciation and knowledge of research continued into the 1980s, which saw the lengthening of midwifery training to 18 months for registered nurses and 3 years for non-nurses to come into line with the European Midwifery Directives. Most of these courses were at diploma or degree level. This, coupled with links to higher education, reinforced the importance of research-based knowledge underpinning midwifery practice.

In 1988 the DHSS funded a midwifery research post as a core post to the NEPU in Oxford. This was a key post and the remit was to undertake and act as a focus for midwifery research. There were few experienced midwife researchers and the establishment of the post created opportunities for support. The NEPU recognized the important contribution that those using the maternity services could make and an effective collaboration was established which has been reflected in many other institutions and initiatives.

The centre also became aware of a great deal of information including a source of untapped skill and research studies pertinent to the care of women and their babies and, with funding from the Department of Health, set up a dedicated midwifery research database (MIRIAD). Its purpose was to assist in the dissemination of findings of ongoing and completed midwifery research studies, thus providing a valuable, easily accessible resource for midwives (MIRIAD was discontinued after the establishment of the National Research Register, see Ch. 4).

Table 7.1 Summary of events/developments impacting on midwifery research

1970s practice and education should be research-based NOT based on tradition or the dictates of others

	Small scale studies	Staffing, role and responsibilities midwife
	Clinical practice	Shaving and enemas research
	Research studentships (DHSS, SHHD scholarships, e.g. Maws educational/Iolanthe Trust	Single projects, dissertations
	DoH funded/longitudinal study (King's College)	Midwives' career prospects
	National Perinatal Epidemiology Unit (NEPU) Oxford	Collaboration midwives/obstetricians
		Computerized pregnancy and childbirth database.
		Cochrane collaboration
1979	DoH funded major study (Chelsea study)	Role and responsibilities of midwife – found underuse of skills, duplication, fragmentation of care

Growing dissatisfaction in midwives and users of the maternity services; need for education

	Advanced Diploma in Midwifery/refresher courses	Emphasis on: research appreciation and research in practice
	Midwifery training period altered 1971	
	Research and the midwife conferences began	Twice per year to disseminate findings
	RCM current awareness bulletin and service	

1980s emphasis on quality and cost-effectiveness as NHS reforms progressed; need for better dissemination of research

	Midwifery training period altered (European Community Directives) 3 years or 18 months for RGN	Expansion of research in curriculum
	Links and moves into higher education	Increase in diplomas and degrees
1988	DoH funded	Midwifery research database MIRIAD
	NEPU publication	Effective Care in Pregnancy and Childbirth
	Midwives Information Digest	MIDIRS
	DoH funded research	Need for direct entry midwife schemes

1990s Era of the consumer, evidence-based practice and clinical effectiveness; also the move from health into higher education for the education of nurses and midwives

	Reports from DoH on R&D National strategy for R&D research and midwifery-specific journals	Government led initiatives to use research results and improve health
		Policy directives about clinical effectiveness and evidence-based care
		Increase in research studies undertaken
1992	DoH English National Board R&D initiatives	Funding focused on specific areas
1993	House of Commons Health Committee	Review maternity services
	Report of Expert Group	Changing Childbirth
1994–1998	Changing childbirth implementation team (CCIT) set up	Take forward initiatives, spread good practice
	Monies for research nationally funded/administered by CCIT	Patterns of care, organization of services, roles, multidisciplinary education, user views and needs
1996	MIDIRS and NHS York centre for reviews	Informed choice leaflets
	Culyer initiative – appointment of research and practice development midwives and nurses in trusts	Research activity identified by trusts
	First Class Service published by DoH	Quality in the NHS document for consultation

Research activity continues to be variable. Dissemination of findings improving but need for staff development. Move into higher education – positive and negative effects on research-based practice

2000 Importance of collaboration emphasized. Government research agenda addressing health inequalities, health economics focusing on cost-effective services

Establishment of National Institute for Clinical Excellence (NICE) to produce guidelines for aspects of treatment and practice. Of relevance to midwives were the *Use of Electronic Fetal Monitoring* (EFM) (NICE 2001a) and *Induction of Labour* (NICE 2001b)

Focus of public health
RCT impact of protocol based midwife-led care in the postnatal period
HOOP trial on perineal care
Focus on birthing centres
Bringing normality into midwifery – Royal College of Midwives (RCM) to set up virtual institute for birth

Shortly after this, in 1989, *A Guide to Effective Care in Pregnancy and Childbirth*, a work containing the systematic reviews on all randomized control trials in pregnancy and childbirth, was published. This has since been re-edited (Enkin et al 2000). The electronic version followed and is now incorporated into the Cochrane pregnancy and childbirth database and is part of the Cochrane Collaboration (http://www.update-software.com/cochrane/). Contained within the paper version is evidence based on trials concerning care and practices. This work is an excellent resource and a good starting point for those involved in the maternity services. It includes recommendations based on the best research evidence available with a list in the appendices of:

- Forms of care that are likely to be beneficial
- Forms of care with a trade-off between beneficial and adverse effects
- Forms of care of unknown effectiveness
- Forms of care unlikely to be beneficial
- Forms of care likely to be ineffective or harmful.

However, the printed version should be used in conjunction with the electronic form (Cochrane Library, Pregnancy and Childbirth Database) which is continually updated as and when new trials are completed. Examples of reviews include:

- Midwife versus medical/shared care
- The effect of social support in pregnancy
- Support from carers during childbirth
- The immediate care of mother and baby
- Postnatal support for breastfeeding women
- Continuity of care.

Although there is a good deal of evidence to support a variety of practices, the Expert Maternity Group (Department of Health 1993) found that tradition and ritual still form the basis for the way in which care is given, with ineffective and unproved practices continuing.

With increased education, greater output of research activity and better sources of dissemination one might be forgiven for thinking that those areas of research known to be of proven value in clinical practice were being implemented and that the profession was developing a research culture. However, an example of a form of care likely to be ineffective or harmful is the routine use of shaving and enemas in labour. We have known this to be the case since the research was conducted some 20 years ago, and it has been publicized in a variety of ways: by publication in a range of journals (Romney 1980, 1982; Romney & Gordon 1981), at midwifery conferences and study events, and by a report in the *Guide to Effective Care in Pregnancy and Childbirth*. Yet the finding in Garcia & Garforth's (1991) study of practices in the maternity services in 1987 found that 16% of units still had a policy of routine enemas and shaving! There is evidence to suggest that the practice continues (Walsh 2001) even though there was a Cochrane update in 2000 supporting previous research (Cuervo et al 2000).

Other examples of ineffective care include antenatal breast or nipple care for women who plan to breastfeed, nipple stimulation tests, electronic fetal monitoring (EFM) without access to fetal scalp sampling during labour, and many more. There have been great strides and it is encouraging that there is evidence of research-based practice but the majority do not see research as being important. The question we need to ask again is why? Research should not become an exercise remote from practice, even for a minority, with many midwives not making the link between research and practice.

THE 1990s: THE ERA OF THE CONSUMER, EVIDENCE-BASED PRACTICE AND CLINICAL EFFECTIVENESS

As we entered the 1990s a number of important changes were taking place in the maternity services which have greatly affected midwives, doctors and women using the service in England. A major catalyst was the government's 1992 review of the maternity services, stimulated by a growing feeling that all was 'not well' with the services being provided. The House of Commons Health Committee (1992) received evidence from users and those providing the maternity services. In their review they stated that 'Becoming a mother is not an illness. It is not an abnormality. It is a normal process' and that there should be control, continuity and choice for those using the services. They also recommended that there should be an expansion of research by midwives, and 'as a matter of priority the Department of Health fund the establishment of extensive pilot schemes in the establishment of midwife managed maternity units within or adjacent to acute hospitals'.

In England the Expert Maternity Group was established to see how this could be achieved and an action plan for purchasers and providers was produced entitled *Changing Childbirth* (Department of Health 1993). This was endorsed and became government policy, being followed up by an executive letter to purchasers (National Health Services Management Executive 1994). Each country in the UK has produced documents relevant to their maternity services but underlying themes include effectiveness and issues of continuity, control and choice (Welsh Office 1992, DHSS Belfast 1994, SHHD 1993). The result of these reports has led to some fundamental changes in the way maternity services are organized with a move towards women being the centre of care.

Empowerment of women means that midwives need to be empowered too and the impact of some of these changes is being researched. In England the establishment by the Department of Health of the changing childbirth implementation team reinforced its commitment to taking these changes forward.

A number of funded projects were developed, involving consumer groups, midwives, doctors and a variety of non-NHS organizations. Projects included a critical appraisal skills programme, to help consumer members of maternity liaison committees to understand and make use of evidence regarding clinical effectiveness, designing a multidisciplinary education system informed by staff and users, and an investigation by the Maternity Alliance of the needs of women with learning difficulties. Many more are researching how care is organized. In view of these changes many trusts began appointing research and practice development midwives. There was a concern about information reaching those who matter – i.e. the users of the service – which has led to a government-funded project on the development of informed choice leaflets produced by MIDIRS and the NHS Centre for Reviews and Dissemination (1996, 1997). For each topic there is a leaflet aimed at users and one for professionals. They are based on what is best practice in the light of available scientific evidence and are an excellent resource but there have been problems within trusts regarding access (Henderson 1996).

Of course the 1990s also saw a plethora of information from the Department of Health following the launch in 1989 of its R&D strategy: *Promoting Clinical Effectiveness* (Department of Health 1996) was launched in 1996; priorities for mothers and children were contained in *Improving the Health of Mothers and Children*, NHS priorities for research (Department of Health 1995); clinical effectiveness was a theme underlying the White Paper outlining the policy for the NHS (Department of Health 1997); and the Green Paper on primary care (Department of Health 1998). However, despite an increase in research activity, much everyday practice is still not evidence-based. The way in which research is approached in the curriculum for future practitioners is critical if research is to underpin the practice of future generations.

Research and the curriculum

Table 7.2 highlights the findings from a telephone survey of five institutions providing midwifery education in 1996 concerning research and the curriculum. They were asked about research teaching, assessment of learning and the perceptions of teachers and students. The institutions surveyed comprised two 'red brick' universities (having a long tradition in research) and three former polytechnics with new university status. They were located in the south-west, south-east, midlands and north. All institutions provided diploma and degree level programmes.

It was reported that at diploma level:

- Research methods as a separate module was inappropriate
- Emphasis should be on the critical appraisal of studies that underpinned practice

Table 7.2 The curriculum and research in 1996 in five midwifery departments*

	A† (new)	B† (rb)	C† (new)	D† (rb)	E† (new)	Comments
Teaching content						
Diploma						
Awareness/appreciation	■	■	■	■	■	Try to instil enthusiasm
Critiquing	■	■	■	■	■	More descriptive than analytical
Simple statistics	■	■	■	■	■	How well this is done varies according to the teacher
Research integral to all other subjects	■	■	■			Number of different teachers to modules/some not midwives/variable as not aware of the midwifery research base
Degree						
Methods in depth	■	■	■	■	■	B Woman-focused research base for care
Advanced statistics	■	■	■	■	■	D Research method shared (120) – small groups midwifery focus
Means of assessment						
Diploma						
Literature review/critique	■		■	■	■	
Degree						
Research proposal				■	■	Process of the proposal development important not outcome
Research study			■	■	■	D Sense of achievement versus credibility/undertaking a piece of research removes fear of research/trust expectation that students do some research
Choice of review or study	■			■		
Statistics paper				■		
Annotated bibliography				■		
In-depth literature review		■				

General comments about teachers' input
Variable confidence/fear of supervision/diploma level less problematic/time commitment problem/teaching load had escalated (especially in newer universities). In both types of university many teachers were also undertaking degrees

Difficulties experienced by students undertaking research studies
Access to clinical areas/shortage of time and support/ethical committee problems

*Universities from four different regions (geographical locations south-east, south-west, midlands, north).
† A, C, E are new universities (new). B and C are 'red brick' universities (rb).

- Other modules in the programme should be based on research evidence.

A report published by the English National Board in 1996 identified that the quality of teaching research was satisfactory but needed continuing development and that those teaching research needed to be involved in it. However, in all five institutions the teaching of research was considered a cause for concern by some teachers and students. Many teachers were undertaking studies themselves and lacked confidence in teaching research as a pure subject or in supervising students undertaking a study. Teaching had become more fragmented as courses became modular with no one to coordinate the whole programme. Ensuring that subjects taught were research based with appropriate midwifery research highlighted was problematic. For students having to carry out a research study anxiety levels increased with issues of seeking permission via ethical and other committees. Other issues raised by students were shortage of time, lack of support and limited access to clinical areas. Some trusts expected students to undertake research; others were of the opinion that the process of research design was important but that the value of undertaking a research study was questioned by both students and teachers. Research in the curriculum should include the whole area of how to integrate research that is known to be beneficial into practice, including the process of change. In an editorial regarding essential components of a course on the utilization of research, Hunt (1996, p. 423) states that: 'The theories of knowledge utilisation and of the management of change became fundamental underpinnings of that course since research utilisation is one form of knowledge utilisation and usually requires some change, be it cognitive or behavioural.' She goes on to emphasize that 'If recognition does not take place within each and every individual who has to put the change into practice it is UNLIKELY TO HAPPEN'.

Since the move of midwifery education away from clinical areas, staff have been limited in their access to resources, for example libraries and information/databases, with reduced teacher contact, once considered of prime importance, particularly in midwifery. Some universities are offering reading and/or borrowing rights, at a price, and most trusts are addressing the issue by providing on-site libraries, but there are difficulties, particularly where there are multiple sites. The educational encounter for midwives, doctors and health professionals is a time when they should learn together. They should be encouraged to question, find, appraise the evidence base of their practice and value the input of those using the service. Above all they should learn together to prepare them to work as part of a team. Educational institutions have improved and are constantly improving all areas of the curriculum and the provision and accessibility of information technology, and support is far better for students today.

THE YEAR 2000 AND BEYOND

The era of health economics and public health: addressing inequalities and more collaborative working between disciplines and agencies providing health and social care

Evidence-based practice and cost-effectiveness continue to be important priorities as we enter the 21st century. To help the effectiveness agenda the government established a National Institute for Clinical Excellence (NICE) (see Chs 2 and 3) and the Commission for Health Improvement (CHI) (Health Services Circular 1998) (see Ch. 4).

NICE has produced two guidelines of relevance to midwives: *The Use of Electronic Fetal Monitoring* (EFM) (NICE 2001a) and *Induction of Labour* (NICE 2001b). However, there are those who argue that to reproduce what we already know is a waste of time and money which should be used to support the development of new evidence (Thornton 2001). In midwifery the drive to bring 'normality' back to midwifery and childbirth and provide woman-centred care continues. Increasing birthing centres is one way that some units are moving forwards while in others midwife-led care is increasing with dedicated areas set aside within consultant units and the midwife as the lead provider. Related to this, within the new healthcare organizations public health has become the focus of intense examination. The midwifery committee of the UKCC commissioned a UK-wide study into the role midwives played in this area (Henderson 2002). The findings demonstrated the complexity and wide-ranging activities in public health in which midwives were involved. It was in those areas that had funded initiatives that were high on the list of priorities for each country where public health activity was greatest. This survey demonstrated that midwives practising in the community work with many groups and should be considered as 'frontline' staff involved in a diversity of practice in respect of public health across the UK.

The Royal College of Midwives (RCM) is in the process of developing an innovative virtual institute for birth that will be a focal point for researchers, midwives, academics, clinical leaders and user organizations both to access and disseminate current research, develop standards for best practice and focus the debate on normal birth. They are bringing together a partnership of organizations, including midwives, academics, health professionals, researchers, user organizations and women, to exchange information, develop partnerships and initiate research into normality in childbirth, both at a local level and globally. By shifting the emphasis back to normality, the virtual institute will seek to ensure that the long-term health of women and children is firmly at the top of the public and political agenda.

This is an area that has been under-funded and under-researched for many years. It became the focus of health technology assessment funding (see Ch. 3) and a randomized control trial was undertaken to assess the impact of midwife-led protocol-based care in the postnatal period and beyond (MacArthur et al 2002). Midwives in the intervention group gave flexible postnatal care tailored to individual needs, while the control group gave standard care. The main effect of the intervention care was a benefit to women's psychological health. Research into the area of the perineum continues (McCandlish et al 2003) and the latest research includes the issue of whether or not to suture, with researchers developing tools to assess the degree of tear in order for midwives to decide (Metcalfe et al 2002).

However, even with a wealth of knowledge into certain aspects of care and the delivery of services, there are still issues that need addressing.

Issues that need to be addressed

Issues that remain to be addressed include dissemination, the skills of appraisal, presentation, managing change and working within an evidence-based culture. If we take note of the research of Hicks (1993), who conducted a survey of midwives' attitudes to, and involvement in, research, we see that she found a significant amount of research activity which had been undertaken by midwives but not published. Midwives perceive research as critical to professional development but lack confidence about the quality of their research and their ability to influence practice.

In *Promoting Clinical Effectiveness* the Department of Health (1996) acknowledges that good access to educational resources, library services and learning events are important. However, there is the implication of time being made available – an expensive commodity. In the real world there is sometimes no time to reflect on practice. It is important to build this into the working week, as the midwife should be involved in the development of protocols underpinning practice. This could be an important part of the UKCC post-registration education and practice (PREP) requirement (which has been adopted by the new Nursing and Midwifery Council which replaced the UKCC in 2002) and critical to adopting guidelines. Ownership is paramount to changing and ensuring that the best possible evidence underpins practice.

The establishment of new systems referred to above will not increase ways of getting research into practice unless other systems are set up to support this. What needs to happen is for clinical units to examine their infrastructure and seek to develop a research culture. Cultures take time to develop and are not easy to change (see Ch. 4) and so it is recognized that a culture that uses research as an integrated part of activity is not easy to develop. There are many useful examples in the nursing literature of frameworks used to promote research-based practice (Kitson et al 1996).

The *Nursing Times Research* journal (NT Research 1998) contains a number of reports and papers of its 1998 symposium proceedings about research-based practice, its practicalities and challenges. In midwifery there is a developing literature about influencing (Renfrew 1997), finding (Hawkins 1998), using (Hicks & Mant 1997) and appraising (Oliver & Needham 1997) the evidence. There are also examples of the practicalities of taking the research agenda forward by increasing research awareness (Hurley 1998, Milne & Hundley 1998). Putting evidence into practice is difficult and needs 'focused intervention in an enabling environment', a point reiterated by Walsh (2001).

In 1998 an evidence-based midwifery network (EBMN) was established as a result of growing concern over getting evidence into practice. Its aim is to enable midwives and user groups to discuss ideas, to network and consider areas that could be usefully explored. The network is supported administratively by the Foundation of Nursing Studies (FoNS) and further details can be found on the FoNS website (http://www.fons.org). It should be noted that at the time of writing concerns about implementation of evidence into practice continue to grow and network membership has grown from 12 to over 480.

As mentioned previously, new structures are being set in place nationally to oversee and monitor the clinical effectiveness agenda. Of equal importance is the need to develop the commitment of those working in trusts. This will not just happen – a local strategy is required. This means bringing a number of differing cultures together, particularly medicine, nursing and midwifery. Success can be determined ultimately where there is a multidisciplinary approach to practice review based on the best evidence available while also taking account of the opinions of those using the service. There follows an account of the initial steps of one women's healthcare unit's attempt to change the midwifery culture of getting research into practice.

THE CLINICAL UNIT AND THE STRATEGY

The project outlined below was given the acronym GRiP as it was designed to 'get research into practice'.

The unit, described as a healthcare trust, is a regional referral unit and has an annual rate of between 5800 and 6200 deliveries and 6000 gynaecological operations. Approximately 4300 births are normal (40 homebirths, no domino scheme). It has a funded whole time equivalent (WTE) establishment of 209 midwives and 150 nurses. The unit is unusual in that it is relatively small and the focus of its activities is specific to neonatal work and women's health. Obstetrics, gynaecology (including oncology) and neonatal services form the basis of the three clinical programmes. At the time of the project there were three advanced nurse practitioners, one supporting each programme, and two lecturer practitioners in midwifery. An initial part of the project was to develop a strategy as there was no identified trust-wide R&D strategy; a database was being established which was primarily concerned with medical research activity. Figure 7.1 diagrammatically represents the proposed strategy for nursing and midwifery which took into account the three main programmes/services provided in the trust. It outlines the infrastructure necessary and sets out the

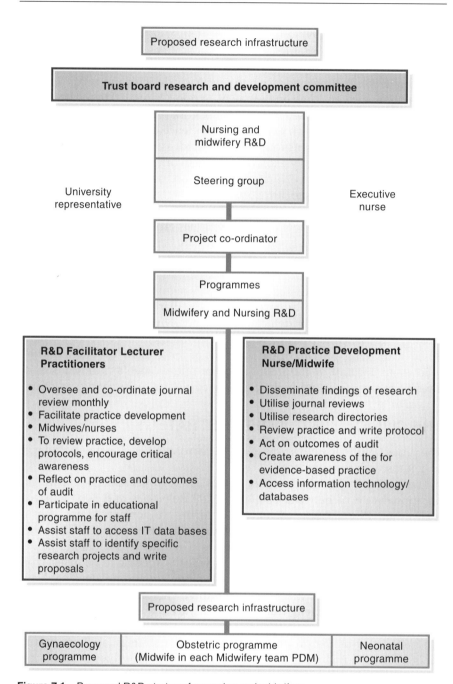

Figure 7.1 Proposed R&D strategy for nursing and midwifery.

responsibilities of the R&D facilitators. The nursing and midwifery steering group feed into the trust R&D committee. Critical to success is the responsibility for R&D being accepted by individuals within each programme. Key roles were discussed at the outset and as the strategy moves forward it is envisaged that changes will be made to take account of developments. The project aims initially were ambitious.

Overall Aims of the GRiP project

- To promote a culture of evidence-based practice by supporting midwives/nurses in understanding research and applying it where appropriate to their practice.
- To encourage and facilitate midwives/nurses to undertake/participate in research that is relevant to this practice and takes cognisance of the trust's corporate research strategy.
- To foster multi-professional collaboration in research.

Objectives and key points

The objectives and the key points to achieving the aims were as follows:

1. *To establish a midwifery/nursing research infrastructure within the trust*

Key points

- Organizational structure/personnel linking clinical units with the university
- Ensuring multi-professional liaison
- Access to information technology and appropriate databases
- Administrative support
- Provision of relevant journals
- Establish a midwifery/nursing research steering group
- Appointment of a research development project leader to spearhead developments.

2. *To develop further the spirit of enquiry and a culture of evidence-based practice*

Key points

- Appointment of a research development facilitator to promote a research culture within the unit
- Determination of a lead nurse/midwife in each directorate/team within the trust to have responsibility for practice developments, protocol review, etc.
- Dissemination of research findings and best practice.

3. *To increase nursing/midwifery research activity especially within the context of multi-professional collaboration within the trust*

4. *To ensure that the direction of midwifery and nursing R&D is integral to the unit's corporate strategy*

Key points

- Establish a database of current research activity/interest
- Conduct a survey of all midwives/nurses to ascertain research knowledge base and skills
- Devise educational activities based on the findings of above
- Determine specific areas of collaboration in line with trust corporate strategy
- Continue an active partnership with the university
- Unit to provide small budget into which staff may bid annually to undertake projects that will promote evidence-based care.

5. *To become recognized nationally for nursing/midwifery R&D in clinical practice*

Key points

- Encourage and foster good publications from midwifery and nursing staff
- Disseminate activities of the staff widely.

The then evidence-based Medical Union within the NHS Executive of the West Midlands provided monies for a person independent of the trust to help facilitate developments. It was recognized that the above aims and objectives would take time to achieve and so the decision was made that the Getting Research into Practice Project (GRiP) would focus only on developing the research-based culture in midwifery.

At the same time as the project was developing the Department of Health launched a clinical effectiveness and research information pack called *Achieving Effective Practice* (Department of Health 1998b). The pack was designed as an education and training resource to support courses and practice-based professional development. It was, and still is, an excellent resource and has been circulated to a wide range of institutions including NHS trusts.

Of course, to be effective and change a culture requires more than well-presented packs of information. The reality of the situation is that there are a number of issues needing to be addressed, for example:

- Stimulating the need to question established practice
- Being able to access information quickly
- Acquiring skills to find and appraise the evidence
- **Then**, being able to take action.

Main phases of the project

Factors contributing to or inhibiting evidence-based activity

The first phase was to identify those factors contributing to or inhibiting evidence-based activity. This involved mapping trust activities, particularly those involving midwives' time, and surveying midwives to find out the experience and skills that the midwives had and to identify any specific development needs to assist individuals in achieving evidence-based practice. Midwives were asked to highlight any perceived barriers and suggest how they might be overcome. What was important was that the project would be linking into existing mechanisms/structures within the trust to achieve its aims as far as possible. Furthermore, collaboration with other groups would be invaluable in helping to foster good interprofessional relationships leading to successful change. It was important to link into other initiatives within the trust, for example a critical appraisal system being introduced by the academic senior registrar which will interface with the GRiP project. The collection of the above information would be invaluable to the second phase although some parts happened simultaneously.

Establishing a model to increase evidence-based activity in midwifery

This involved developing a robust communication strategy that was practical and user-friendly. It also involved identifying from the survey exactly what were the staff development needs as perceived by the midwives themselves. There was also opportunity for midwives to nominate themselves to form practice review groups. These groups were to be key in looking at real questions arising from midwifery practice at that time and in that unit, and therefore relevant to midwives.

Summary of survey results mentioned in phase one

The survey was conducted to determine:

- The extent of research and related activities currently being undertaken by midwives
- The barriers that may be hindering staff in utilizing evidence in practice
- The educational needs of midwives in achieving clinical effectiveness.

A response rate of 63% was achieved, with 123 questionnaires out of a total 194 being returned. Forty-six midwives in the sample were graded G (37%), 40 graded F (33%), 33 graded E (27%) with 4 (3%) midwives on a higher grading. The sample was evenly spread between full-time, 63 (51%), and part-time, 57 (46%). Over half of staff (60%) had been qualified between 4 and 20 years with the overall mean being 12.5 years. Of the total sample, 25 (20%) midwives were participating in research studies; most of these were locally managed or regional studies and three were nationally managed. Research being undertaken by four midwives related to their degree studies.

Midwives were or had been involved in a range of research related activities; many were enthusiastic and had changed their practice as a result of research findings and audit. Reasons for non-attendance (by 96% of the sample) at the researchers ruminations group (the group that discussed all research projects in the unit and decided if they should go ahead) included not being aware of the group, being released from clinical areas, and time constraints. Although 86 (70%) midwives agreed that protocols and guidelines supported the implementation of evidence-based practice in the trust, 37 (30%) midwives did not agree. Midwives stated that some guidelines were out of date, some were unworkable, others had no evidence source and midwives were excluded from their development even though they affected their practice. There is a need for a process for reviewing guidelines and protocols on a regular basis. Involvement of all groups of staff is critical to the implementation of evidence-based practice.

Barriers to activities related to evidence-based practice were divided into three areas:

- Organizational factors to do with time, support, access to and resources available
- Lack of cooperation between and with people, particularly medical staff
- The volume of research and the difficulty in appraising it.

It is clear from comments made that many midwives in the sample were confident in making decisions about practice in the light of evidence and women's wishes. However, there are a number who lack confidence and would benefit from support and/or education in developing the skills associated with evidence-based practice. On conclusion of the project two main recommendations were put forward (see below).

Recommendations to the unit

The following recommendations were made to the unit:

1. Support to develop and coordinate evidence-based practice in midwifery and nursing

Fulfilment of this would help to address issues to do with barriers. This could be achieved by:

- Identifying key people in each programme to be *actively* responsible for evidence-based activity in nursing and midwifery so that developments are not ad hoc and there is coordination across the trust. This should include the establishment of a multi-professional forum for developing and reviewing guidelines concerning midwifery and nursing practice. It should also include appropriate skill development of staff.

- The appointment of a nurse or midwife to the R&D centre in the trust. This person could provide support for midwives wishing to undertake research and research-related activities. Currently the trust is missing opportunities for generating income, which it could capitalize on if adequate support were available. The introduction of such a post would also assist cooperation and collaboration within and between professional groups.

2. Expansion and development of resources available

Implementing clinical effectiveness is a resource-intensive activity. While knowing how to use the resources available is important, easy access is also critical. There should be:

- One computer per clinical area. As the hospital network expands, *all* staff should benefit. Suggestions made by midwives about the network and guidelines for practice should be seriously considered.
- A centrally based database to capture the work undertaken on courses. The trust expends a great deal of money supporting midwives pursuing further academic studies. The collection of evidence related to clinical activity is being undertaken but there appears to be no formal record of the detail from which all groups of staff may benefit.
- A central register of all research and research related activities of all professional groups in the trust.

Possible solutions to many of the issues raised by midwives are contained in the main report (Henderson 1999).

SUMMARY AND CONCLUSION

This chapter has looked briefly at midwifery research from the 1970s to the present, its organization and focus. It has also raised issues that are still relevant today, particularly those of implementation of evidence into practice. An example of a strategy was included which was part of a project carried out in 1998 to get evidence into practice. The phases of the project were described. Within the project there were a number of issues raised which required action. These were to do with staff and skill development, time for research and/or evidence-based activities, availability and use of resources and the process and involvement in developing protocols and guidelines. Coordination and support for these activities are critical. It is important to note the perception by midwives of 'how it is' and that they are committed to moving the clinical governance agenda, including evidence-based practice, forward. Changes were made as a result of the project and attitudes did change.

Further developments were supported by the appointment of a clinically based research nurse. However, to change a culture is to change the way people think and behave and that takes continuing time, energy and commitment. A strategy is required that is supported by all groups (including users) and all professions but most of all there needs to be a willingness on the part of everyone to continue to be committed, to cooperate and to collaborate. These are essential to success. People matter – they need to feel valued, be made aware of the existence of the evidence, and feel that it is important before they will alter their practice. We would do well to remember that: 'He who is forced to change against his will is of his own opinion still' (anon). If this is the case then it will be reflected in the care that is given, which may not be the most beneficial. Research-based practice has been part of our language and, for many, the basis of practice for a number of years and yet it seems that in some ways we have not moved forward. In the words of Winston Churchill: 'This is not the end, it is not even the beginning of the end, it is the end of the beginning.'

REFERENCES

Changing Childbirth Implementation Team (CCIT) 1996 Maternity service liaison committees. Department of Health, London

Cuervo L, Roderiguez M, Delgado M 2000 Enemas during labour. Cochrane review. Cochrane Library, issue 4, Update Software, Oxford

Department of Health and Social Security 1972 Report of the Committee on Nursing (chaired by Asa Briggs) Cmnd 5115. HMSO, London

Department of Health 1993 Report of the Expert Maternity Group chaired by Baroness Cumberledge, vol. 1: Changing childbirth. HMSO, London

Department of Health 1995 Improving the health of mothers and children. NHS Executive, London

Department of Health 1996 Promoting clinical effectiveness. NHS Executive, London

Department of Health 1998a First class service: quality in the NHS. NHS Executive, London

Department of Health 1998b Achieving effective practice. NHS Executive, London

Department of Health and Social Services Belfast 1994 Delivering choice: midwife and GP led maternity units. Report of the Northern Ireland Maternity Units Study Group. Department of Health, Belfast

ENB 1996 Teaching research in nursing and midwifery curriculum. Occasional Report. English National Board for Nursing, London

Enkin M, Keirse M, Neilson J et al 2000 A guide to effective care in pregnancy and childbirth, 3rd edn. Oxford University Press, Oxford

Garforth S, Garcia J 1991 Admitting a weakness or a strength. Midwifery 3: 10–24

Hawkins M 1998 Finding the evidence: a guide to information sources. British Journal of Midwifery 6(4): 215–219

Health Services Circular 1998/021 Better health and better health care. Department of Health, London

Henderson C 1996 Prioritising the priorities: is there a choice? British Journal of Midwifery 4(3): 117–119

Henderson C 1999 Evidence based practice and the Birmingham Women's Healthcare NHS Trust. Final report for partnership for developing quality (PDQ). West Midlands NHS Executive, Birmingham

Henderson C 2002 The midwifery contribution to public health in the United Kingdom, November 2001–February 2002. University of Birmingham, Birmingham

Hicks C 1992 Research in midwifery: are midwives their own worst enemies? Midwifery 8: 2–18

Hicks C 1993 A survey of midwives attitudes to, and involvement in, research: the first stage in identifying needs for a staff development programme. Midwifery 9: 51–62

Hicks N, Mant J 1997 Using the evidence: putting research into practice. British Journal of Midwifery 5(7): 396–399

House of Commons Health Committee 1992 Review of the maternity services, chaired by Sir Nicholas Winterton. HMSO, London

Hunt J 1996 Barriers to research utilisation [editorial]. Journal of Advanced Nursing 23: 423–425

Hurley J 1998 Midwives and research based practice. British Journal of Midwifery 6(5)

Kitson A, Bana A, Harvey G, Thompson D 1996 From research to practice: one organisational model for promoting research based practice. Journal of Advanced Nursing Practice 23: 430–440

MacArthur C, Winter H R, Bick D et al 2002 Redesigning postnatal care: a randomised controlled trial of protocol-based midwifery-led care focussed on individual women's physical and psychological health needs. Health Technology Assessment. [Available from the National Coordinating Centre for Health Technology Assessment (email hta@soton.ac.uk) or off the web at http://www.ncchta.org]

McCandlish R, Renfrew M, Kettle C, Garcia J, Bowler U 2003 The HOOP study: robust evidence for perineal care? British Journal of Midwifery 11(3): 143–147

Metcalfe A, Tohill S, Williams A, Haldon V, Brown L 2002 A pragmatic tool for the measurement of perineal tears. British Journal of Midwifery 10(7): 412–417

MIDIRS and the NHS Centre for Reviews and Dissemination 1996 and 1997 Informed Choice Leaflets. 1996 Series 1 Support in labour. Fetal heart rate monitoring in labour. Ultrasound screening. Alcohol in pregnancy. Positions in labour and delivery. 1997 Series 2 Epidurals. Breastfeeding or bottlefeeding. Antenatal screening for congenital abnormalities. Breech presentation. Place of birth. MIDIRS, 9 Elmdale Road, Clifton, Bristol BS8 1SL, UK. Freephone 0800 581009

Milne J, Hundley V 1998 A strategy for raising research awareness among midwives. British Journal of Midwifery 6(6): 374–378

National Health Services Management Executive 1994 Purchasing priorities 1994–1995. EL (94)9. Department of Health, London

National Institute for Clinical Excellence 2001a The use of electronic fetal monitoring. Inherited clinical guideline C, May 2001. National Institute for Clinical Excellence, London

National Institute for Clinical Excellence 2001b Induction of labour. Inherited clinical guideline D, June 2001. National Institute for Clinical Excellence, London

Nursing Times Research 1998 Focus on research based practice. Reports and papers from a symposium. 3(1)

Oliver S, Needham G 1997 Continuity of carer: what can we learn from a Cochrane Review? British Journal of Midwifery 5(5): 292–295

Renfrew M 1997 Influencing the development of evidence-based practice. British Journal of Midwifery 5(3): 131–134

Romney M L 1980 Predelivery shaving: an unjustified assault? Journal of Obstetrics and Gynaecology 1: 33–35

Romney M L, Gordon H 1981 Is your enema really necessary? British Medical Journal 282: 1269–1271

Romney M L 1982 Nursing research in obstetrics and gynaecology. International Journal of Nursing Studies 19(4): 193–203

Sackett D L, Richardson W S, Rosenberg W, Haynes R B 1997 Evidence-based medicine: how to practice and teach EBM. Churchill Livingstone, New York

Scottish Home and Health Department 1993 Provision of maternity services in Scotland – a policy review. HMSO, Edinburgh

Thomson A, Robinson S 1985 Dissemination of midwifery research: how this has been facilitated in the UK. Midwifery 1: 52–53

Thornton J 2001 Not so NICE clinical guidelines. British Journal of Midwifery 9(8): 470–472

Walsh D 2001 And finally … how do we put all the evidence into practice? British Journal of Midwifery 9(2): 74–80

Welsh Office 1992 The protocol for investment in health gain. HMSO, Cardiff

IMPORTANT WEBSITES

http://www.update-software.com/cochrane/
http://www.nelh.nhs.uk/midwife/Default.asp
This site gives access to a number of important sites relating to evidence-based practice and policies affecting practice.
http://www.nice.org.uk/catlist.asp
http://www.chi.nhs.uk/
http://www.doh.gov.uk/nsf/

8

Experiences in children's nursing practice

Jane Coad   Liz Morgan

with contributions from Chris Holden and Joy Grech

Editors' comment

This chapter examines work completed in a childcare setting. In focusing on the simple yet essential idea of information-gathering and collation in the form of a database, it offers useful insights into what can be described as the first step in developing research at an organizational level. Lack of awareness of the range of research activity in any organization means, at one level, that the last vital step of dissemination has not been developed. At another level, it could mean that there is unnecessary duplication of effort, one of the key reasons for developing an R&D strategy (see Ch. 2). The clinical examples included in the chapter were identified through the database and not only offer good examples of the nature of research work that can be carried out but also highlight the need for a clear strategy for sharing research activities.

INTRODUCTION

Within healthcare settings the process for ensuring the safety of patients and minimizing the risk of untoward incidents is increasingly important. From this perspective, it is important that nurses build an evidence base to support and extend their understanding of the impact of the care they deliver. In this way, for example, nurses can question the effectiveness of long-established practices. Many of these enhance the care and well-being of patients. However, there may be other practices that provide no real value to the patient experience (Department of Health 2000). Indeed, some serve as an obstacle to change and 'new ways of working' that really would improve the quality and efficiency of patient care.

With these perspectives in mind, this chapter will outline one initiative with examples from clinical practice in children's nursing. We will seek to demonstrate that research directly related to patient care can be undertaken in the everyday clinical setting. The ability to critically analyse situations and respond rapidly to the evidence is a key skill in our technical world where the speed at which healthcare is delivered is ever increasing. Nurses are very adept at working in such an environment, and capable of making complex decisions in the best interests of patients and their families.

It has been suggested that there is a reluctance to transfer these skills from the bedside to what they perceive as the academic world in which research is undertaken (Walsh 1997). This is being addressed in that most nursing education courses, in common with all other health professions (see Ch. 6) now include opportunity for nurses to study research methodology as a core component of the curriculum. It is important therefore to ask why there remains such a challenge to nurses and other healthcare professions to undertake and publish research (HEFCE 2001).

The reasons for the difficulties experienced in encouraging nurses to use research are multifaceted (Funk et al 1991). However, easy access to information is vital. It is true that the transition of nursing education into higher education institutions in England, for example, did impact for a short time on the availability of library resources in hospitals. Another factor thought to contribute to nurses' reluctance to use research is a lack of confidence in their ability to critically appraise research literature. Many nurses still feel uncomfortable with their research skills for the reason noted above, i.e. it is something for 'academics' to do. Therefore it is essential to target these groups of staff with a programme of continuing professional development (CPD) to enhance these skills.

One of the challenges lies in the emphasis on delivering clinical care in an environment in which, for example, there are many targets set by the Department of Health (Department of Health 2003). This creates competing demands on time in which managerial objectives must be met. While care management issues are essential, it is important to consider ways in which, in such managerially orientated environments, research can contribute to the development of better care and subsequently to maintenance of standards, staff development, recruitment and retention of a committed, motivated workforce.

The question, however, remains – how can organizations encourage research? A crucial factor is leadership, commitment and support from senior managers in both a visionary and a practical sense. Staff need firstly the encouragement to develop an understanding of research methodology, tools and techniques and subsequently the opportunity to apply this knowledge and skill. One way of doing this is to undertake small studies in the first instance to build confidence. Furthermore, it has been suggested that implementing research findings does not appear to come naturally to nurses. Initially, this was because this was a new concept, but the body of knowledge developed by nurses about the effectiveness of some nursing practice has increased and yet there remains a failure to modify practice in the light of the findings and recommendations.

It is important that nurses do respond and implement research findings as appropriate. However, it is acknowledged that this is not a simple process as the skills involved in critiquing research evidence are high level skills which demand both high level research knowledge (Chs 1 and 12) and the managerial skills required to effect organizational change (see Ch. 4).

Active encouragement for nurses to study research methodology should be a part of the portfolio for lifelong learning in clinical care settings. Small studies can be encouraged through supporting staff to undertake higher degrees while larger studies are probably more successful if developed as a collaborative venture between clinical units and their local university (Ch. 2). From small beginnings there are opportunities available for nurses to apply for research funding to facilitate larger studies, which in turn can lead to the dissemination of findings, which will in turn serve to influence current practice.

Peer support

An important element of any development opportunity is peer support, and therefore consideration should be given to ways of providing this. One way is to establish a 'research interest' or journal group where individual members of staff involved in research activities can seek advice and guidance from colleagues. To do this it is necessary to find out what people are doing. Sharing knowledge of activities is one step in the process of developing a research orientated environment. Establishing a directory or database of staff research experience, expertise and interests is key to the process of exploring ways in which knowledge and skill can be shared.

CURRENT ISSUES IN CHILD HEALTH RESEARCH

The importance of research-based nursing practice is enshrined in the 5-year nursing strategy, at one children's hospital. To achieve this goal staff have been supported to undertake research awareness courses and studies have been supported by development of a good resource base that includes investment in relevant journals and CD-ROM databases, for example the Cochrane Library (see Ch. 4). The opportunity to establish a multidisciplinary education centre and library was taken as part of the hospital development so the issue of this resource was addressed. The hospital has a proactive multi-professional research and development (R&D) strategy that supports both research development and dissemination. Seminars and local study days relating to developing research in child health are regular features and these enable nurses to share work that has been undertaken and from which others may wish to learn. However, despite such advances there remained a need for nursing staff to learn more about nursing research activities across the trust.

THE NURSING RESEARCH DATABASE

To overcome some of the previously outlined issues, a nursing research development group was formed in 1997 (Coad et al 2001). This was given the name PRAM (paediatric research action members). This group is jointly coordinated by a member of the lecturing staff from a local university and the professional development team at the hospital. The initiation and development of this database will be outlined below.

The overall aim of the PRAM group project is: 'To support the research strategy through the development of a directory of information and nursing research activities/experience within the Children's Hospital NHS Trust, which is accessible and user-friendly to all staff.'

Establishing the group

At the first meeting the PRAM group members noted they were unclear about which nurses had undertaken or were currently undertaking research projects within the hospital. The group wanted to know who had done and who was doing research and how to contact them across the hospital but felt that they often learned about projects through an informal, ad hoc route. Thus, as the nursing strategy was being developed, the coordinators, with senior management support, felt that this would be an ideal opportunity to develop a research directory stored on a database within the education centre of the hospital but accessible to all staff in the clinical units.

To achieve this goal the project team requested each ward/unit across the trust to identify a link coordinator to collect data from each member of qualified nursing staff related to their academic and practical experience of research. The link representatives were drawn from each clinical area and included staff from the community and special school settings who worked closely with the hospitals.

This group meets regularly to discuss new developments and initiatives. In some areas, it was felt that two members of staff would be more effective due to the number of staff involved and to act as 'buddies' to one another, thus covering all the meetings and subsequent support. Indeed, in the case of the paediatric intensive care unit (PICU), where the nursing staff complement is over 140, four group members currently support one another and work as active members sharing the project. As the existing members grow in confidence and skills they also act as buddies to new members unfamiliar with the group dynamics and the complexities of project fieldwork.

It was agreed that in order for the momentum of the project to be maintained regular meetings must take place. Both hospital and university management fully supported the project and the time spent on the collection and collation of the database is viewed as essential academic/clinical liaison work (see Ch. 6).

From the outset, it was decided that meetings would be informal and open to all grades of staff. Honesty was also seen as an important principle so that participating staff could raise any concerns. The group felt this was an approachable 'top-down/bottom-up' framework in which feedback of information to education and clinical staff would be understandable and would ultimately enhance the success of the project.

Action plan

One of the first steps was to devise a structured action plan. Using an action plan approach the group set out realistic time spans and achievable goals to work from. In order to collect the data a simple, open questionnaire was devised using a face-to-face interview tool, which could be used in a one-to-one or focus group interview approach (Table 8.1). Interview training was undertaken with the coordinators and, after the pilot study, modifications were made to the semi-structured questionnaire.

It was felt that a flexible tool with open-ended questions would be the most successful in eliciting the required information. Each member of nursing staff was asked to voluntarily provide information about their research activities and experience. There was a lot of support for this project and everyone approached has been willing to share their experience in the

Table 8.1 The PRAM interview schedule*

Outline of the interview schedule for the paediatric research action members (PRAM) database
1. Name
2. What is the area in which you currently work? (Include ward/dept/community/address)
3. Have you undertaken any research courses including research modules, courses, projects and/or study days? *(Prompt – what? Subject/title/any details i.e. nursing or multidisciplinary, type of courses or research based activity?)*
4. Have you undertaken any research projects? *(Prompt – details such as when with whom or by self and role? Include type of activity/skills e.g. bid writing/report writing)*
5. Would you like to participate in any research activities in the future? *(Prompt – such as expand on course requirements and interests)*
6. Is there any other information that you would like us to know?
Interviewer signature..

*Copyright to JCLM/PRAMBCH03

format described. This is an immense challenge for group members as currently the nursing establishment is over 750 whole-time equivalents. Following completion of this process, a user-friendly research directory was compiled for all staff to access.

Developing the initiative

The PRAM group continued to grow! Meetings were advertised through various channels such as posters in clinical units, discussion at the key meetings attended by nurses within the hospital, use of the hospital computer link-up and direct telephone calls. Beyond the hospital some of the link coordinators presented their work at several national nursing conferences using posters and slides.

As with many other groups, the challenge was to maintain the initiative. Using a SWOT analysis (see Chs 4 and 5) the group were able to identify and address many important issues pertaining to the project (Table 8.2). In order to overcome the issues identified in Table 8.2, an inbuilt programme of training for the data collectors was organized and ongoing information has been widely published across the trust to reduce any anxieties. Thus to date no nurse has refused to be interviewed and protection of their data is paramount as we develop the database further.

As outlined, developing research in practice can also be difficult, particularly given the continuing and rapid nature of change within the National Health Service (Bradshaw 1995). One problematic issue is also the cost of such a group. However, it is interesting to note that the tangible financial costs were under £100, but what is immeasurable is the time and energy each member has contributed to the group. However, the opportunity of developing the database, particularly in the new climate of an evolving nursing strategy and an increased emphasis on evidence-based care as part of the R&D strategy, was important. The potential to make a strong impact on clinical care as a result of informing the staff of evidence available was seen as immense.

Data protection

Initially, the clinical nurses in the group did not have the necessary skills related to building up such a large database of information. Such skills were therefore recruited from within the secretarial support of the education centre at the trust. This assistance has been invaluable in storing and retrieving the vital information. However, at the same time a programme of database information seminars has been organized to help group members to build up their knowledge. A database format using Microsoft Access has been devised to load the nursing information.

One logistical issue was how to protect the information provided by the participants and subsequent updating of the database. It was decided that

Table 8.2   SWOT analysis of the PRAM group

Strengths	Weaknesses
• Group of dedicated nurses with one aim; to find out and improve research awareness of activities across the trust • The innovative leadership model of linking the trust and one university has successfully bridged theory and practice within the clinical environment • Academic and clinical nurses/forging closer links to network and share information • Development of a research 'user friendly' directory that is accessible to all staff • Acknowledgement of each individual contribution to the team • Establishment of a 'buddy' system to aid support • Identification of nursing research within the hospital and the university • Established programme to develop nursing research skills for all members • Acknowledgement of 'nurturing' and supporting the researchers of the future	• Limited interview skills and database training of group members at the start of the project • The issue of confidentiality was of paramount concern; for staff to consent to this project they must be given the assurance that the information collected would be safeguarded and only accessed for its identified purpose. Data protection therefore had to be addressed, concluding that the research directory should only be available through a gatekeeper • Acknowledgement of enormity of inputting and updating data • Limited resources available
Opportunites	Threats
• The development of research skills and confidence, therefore enhancing the profile of the trust • Development and sharing of research skills and knowledge • Presentation of group activities and promotion of the advantages of linking NHS trusts and universities to bridge theory and practice. Examples of this include conference presentations and publications • Vision for the future. Link other nursing, medical and allied multi-professional databases together • Contribute to the regional and national picture of paediatric research activities	• Timescale, e.g. interview time had to be extended, due to constraints and training issues • Time constraints as each member of the group has full-time work commitments; therefore time for collection and collation of information by questionnaire required negotiation with clinical managers and also individual dedication • Accessibility of data • Financial support

to ensure protection of data a 'gatekeeper' role would be needed. It was intended that this person would act as a 'protector' to the nursing research information and would not give out details until the person who 'owned' the data was approached and had consented.

There were concerns surrounding the question of who the 'gatekeeper' would be and how this would be organized. This has been resolved by working with key personnel within the education centre at the hospital. Consequently, while all staff can read and visit the database for information, the gatekeepers are the only staff with the access to edit any aspects of the database.

Future directions

To date, the group has completed the process of data collection and collation of the staff has taken place ($n = 750$ whole-time equivalents). The challenge now is that the database requires additional manpower to keep it updated.

Staff have been kept up to date about the database through regular correspondence, the continuation of the regular PRAM meetings and clear leadership model, and presentations at every opportunity across the trust. These have even included an official 'launch day' with balloons and free food for staff!

The PRAM group feel that joint participation between the university and clinical areas serves to facilitate the linking of theory to practice (Coad et al 2001). This has meant that lecturing staff in education and clinical staff in the hospital trust can be rallied to generate additional interest and support for the project. Research skills are being developed within the group through the networking of research-based knowledge and experience. In the future it is intended that through this database potential research projects will be identified. Preliminary discussions with healthcare and academic colleagues have taken place with a view to developing a broader multi-professional perspective, which will enhance the database even further. Indeed, most recently two national research bids have been applied for.

PROJECTS IDENTIFIED

As a result of the PRAM database project a number of different projects were identified in the hospital. To illustrate this, two clinical research exemplars are outlined below. The PRAM database had drawn this work out from local activity and made the information more widely available to clinical staff thus demonstrating the value of a database making research more accessible to others. Sharing of information in a relatively straightforward way could be seen to have tangible benefits.

Exemplar 8.1   Psychological preparation for nasogastric feeding in children

Chris Holden, Nutritional Care Clinical Nurse Specialist

Summary

The research project explored the psychological preparation for children requiring nasogastric feeding and involved collaboration from dietetic, nursing, play therapist, statistician and senior medical colleagues. Funding for clerical support was made available by the author obtaining a Portex scholarship from the Association of British Paediatric Nursing (ABPN).

Literature review

It has long been recognized that children and parents require preparation and support in the event of hospitalization (Melamed & Ridley-Johnson 1988, Glasper et al 1992). Programmes that prepare children for hospitalization are designed to inform the child about what will happen and to familiarize the child with the hospital environment (Hunsberger et al 1994). Information about healthcare procedures can be provided through modelling, procedural and sensory information, and repeated information and support (Holden & MacDonald 2000).

Some studies have evaluated the effectiveness of distraction techniques that have proved useful in reducing a child's pain and behavioural distress during an acute experience (Vessey et al 1994). It is well documented that therapeutic play is the ideal way to prepare children for procedures (Abbott 1990, Boatwright & Crummette 1991). Rope & Bush (1994) have received the psychological preparation for paediatric oncology patients undergoing painful procedures and commented on its effectiveness. Ellerton et al (1994) reviewed the coping behaviour of 80 pre-school children during venepuncture. They suggest that a child's coping is related to the situation and the actions of professionals in that situation rather than to the characteristics of the individual child.

Boliq et al (1991) report that medical play and preparation have become increasingly visible components of psychosocial programming for children in healthcare settings. Medical play and preparation represent different philosophies and theories of children's learning, adaptation and development. Jay (1988) emphasizes four basic types of intervention to decrease distress and increase coping skills in children undergoing invasive medical procedures, namely preparation, hypnosis, behaviour therapy, and cognitive behavioural interventions.

Psychological preparation is thought to be helpful in reducing stress in paediatric patients undergoing surgery (Boliq et al 1991, Mansson et al 1992). However, literature pertaining to preparation for enteral feeding was found to be limited (Young 1994). A pilot study carried out at the Birmingham Children's Hospital NHS Trust explored children's experiences of enteral feeding. This pilot elicited conflicting views about the need for psychological preparation for nasogastric feeding and concluded that children should be given the choice of whether or not to receive information and preparation (Holden et al 1997). This study therefore sought to redress this balance.

Method

The aim of the study was to test the hypothesis that enterally fed children who receive detailed psychological preparation before feeding, and continuing supportive care subsequently, are less upset by the experience of nasogastric feeding than children who receive standard, low-intensity preparation and support. Ethical approval was sought and obtained for this study.

Psychological preparation of children undergoing enteral nutrition by nasogastric tube was evaluated in a prospective study of 48 children nursed at home. They were randomly allocated to receive either standard informal preparation or detailed psychological preparation and support. The children were divided into two groups according to age: group A comprised toddlers and younger children aged 2–6 years and group B comprised older children and adolescents aged 7–16 years. Questionnaires were administered to all parents and older children by dietetic colleagues who were blinded to the type of preparation received by the children.

Findings

This was the first study to examine the role of the preparation of children for nasogastric feeding. However, results need to be interpreted with caution because of the small sample size.

Results emphasized that detailed psychological preparation of families takes time. Routine preparation and psychological support appeared to be beneficial for older children but the passage of a nasogastric tube was seen as very distressing to both parents and children. Having a nasogastric tube was perceived as a major problem specifically by group A. There was no statistical difference in the effects of enteral nutrition between younger children who received routine preparation and those who received detailed preparation; however, parental assessment of their child's behaviour was the sole means of determining how the younger child felt and reacted.

In group B, there were marked differences: scores suggested that those who received detailed preparation had been better prepared for enteral feeding in hospital and at home and that the passage of the nasogastric tube, although unpleasant, was less distressing to them ($P < 0.05$). Talking to nurse and play therapist was seen by parents as essential ($P < 0.05$). The authors conclude that children should be prepared for painful procedures and followed up sensitively, according to their needs.

Published literature in the form of a patient information booklet was developed from this study incorporating the views and opinions of adolescents who had undertaken nasogastric feeding. The booklet provides important information about the advantages and disadvantages of nasogastric feeding. The questionnaire data have also improved understanding of how tube feeding is likely to affect the child's day-to-day activities. Information about problems, eating orally, getting on with friends, sleeping at night with the pump and going to the toilet frequently are all now discussed in detail.

Talking with nurses and play therapists was considered extremely important. Parents thought that repetition of the information and continued support is essential. The study data support the notion that detailed psychological preparation of families by all members of the team takes time. Research addressing the issue of children undergoing painful/distressing procedures needs to be developed by psychologists, nursing staff and play therapists.

Overall, the study report improved the team's understanding of the child's perception of his/her illness, his/her cognitive development, and the illness concepts required when supporting families and children. Thus, children should be well prepared and followed up carefully and sensitively to help prevent adverse psychological consequences. While the findings must be interpreted with caution in view of the small sample size of older children, it was encouraging to find that this group were helped by careful preparation and supportive care.

Implications for practice

As a result of this project specific changes were made to care. These included:

- Every child should be individually assessed so that effective support can be given to parents/carers and children. At BCH NHS Trust, it is now routinely requested that the play therapist is involved in pre- and post-procedural preparation of children undergoing nasogastric tube feeding.
- The need for interdisciplinary working is essential in feeding problems. Currently, the parent, play therapist, psychologist, nurse or whoever is teaching the technique undertakes a plan of care which includes the children's views and feelings, thus helping them to help themselves.

Exemplar 8.2   Parents' perceptions of family needs in a paediatric intensive care unit

Joy Grech, Research Nurse, Paediatric Intensive Care Unit

Summary

This exemplar describes a study developed in order to explore the needs of the family of the critically ill child in a lead centre paediatric intensive care unit (PICU). There is little previous research into the needs of parents with a child in paediatric intensive care (PIC) in the UK and this was felt to be important information in caring for this group of children and their families.

Literature review

PIC in the UK is currently undergoing reorganization resulting in the establishment of lead centres, following the guidelines made within the two most recent reports (Department of Health 1997a, 1997b). Recommendations for the care of the family of the critically ill child made within these reports include:

- Orientation to the unit
- An explanation that parents can have continual access to their child
- Introduction to key members of the PIC team
- Encouragement to interact physically and verbally with their child
- Encouragement to express feelings and concerns
- Referral to community agencies
- Help in preparing themselves and the family for the possible death or only partial recovery of their child.

The majority of studies examining family needs in PIC are small-scale, quantitative in design, and have concentrated on parental needs. Many of the studies have relied on Molter's (1979) Critical Care Family Needs Inventory

(CCFNI) tool, although adaptations to the tool for use in paediatrics have been made (Farrel & Frost 1992, Fisher 1994). In summary, previous research has identified the most important needs of the family with a child in PIC as:

- Honest, understandable and regular information about the patient's treatment, progress, changes and diagnosis
- To be with the child
- To feel that the hospital staff care about the child
- To be assured that the child is receiving the best possible care.

For the majority of parents in PIC, the main concern is the recovery of their child. Although it would appear from previous studies that patient-related needs outweigh family-related needs and concerns, this does not mean that family needs are of no importance. Indeed, a major part of the paediatric nurse's role involves caring for parents (Callery 1997). PIC nurses must help parents to support their child in critical care in order to maintain the parent child/relationship (Fisher 1994). No research studies to date have examined the specific needs of the culturally and socially diverse families likely to be cared for in a lead centre in the UK, in addition to which little attention has been paid to the needs of children who stay in PIC long-term. The roles and experiences of other family members have also received scant attention in the research literature, and these issues will be explored from the parents' perspective in this study. Noyes (1998) suggests that the way forward for research into parental needs in PIC is to adopt a qualitative approach, thus exploring family needs from a 'holistic insider perspective'. This study will adopt this perspective in order to explore family needs in the PICU. There is currently a lack of evidence available to guide practice in the care of all families of children in PIC.

Aims of the study

The aim of the study was to explore parents' perceptions of the needs of the family with a child in a lead centre PICU.

Method

A phenomenological study was undertaken using semi-structured interviews with parents of children following discharge from the PICU. The following parents were excluded from the study:

- Parents of children who were subject to child protection procedures
- Parents whose children had died
- Parents who filed a formal complaint while their child was in hospital.

Data were collected over a period of approximately 2 weeks, with a total of 24 semi-structured interviews. Interviewing parents at what is usually a stressful and anxiety-provoking time required great sensitivity (Lee 1993). Parents were given a verbal explanation and a written information sheet at least 24 hours before they were asked to participate in the study.

It was originally intended to include those parents whose first language was not English. Due to operational difficulties this will now be carried out as a separate study. Interviews were taped and analysed using a phenomenological approach in order to identify family needs from a healthcare 'user perspective'.

Permission to conduct the study was obtained from the PIC clinical director, clinical nurse manager. A summary of the project proposal was circulated to all managers and consultants of the wards to which patients could have been transferred following their PICU stay. All research participants were assured of anonymity at all times. Ethical approval was obtained from the research ethics group. Parents were aware that they could withdraw from the study at any time, without reason, and that this would not affect the care of their child in any way.

Before commencing the interview, the interviewer stressed to parents that the care of their child would not be affected if they refused to participate, and that they could terminate the interview, without having to give a reason, at any point. Parents were asked if they wished some comments to be relayed anonymously to appropriate persons; for example security issues raised were already being addressed by the PIC manager. The semi-structured interviews were piloted with three parents prior to the main data collection period. Interviews were taped, and demographic data were collected before the interview. Tapes were kept in a locked cupboard. Only members of the research team had access to the tapes. On completion of the study, the tapes were to be destroyed.

Data analysis

Interview tapes were transcribed and checked for validity by the project team. Common themes were extracted, as suggested by Colaizzi (1978). A sample of these are presented below.

Findings

As indicated in Figure 8.1, the interview sample was broken down into mothers, fathers and couples. Mothers were the largest group of those being interviewed.

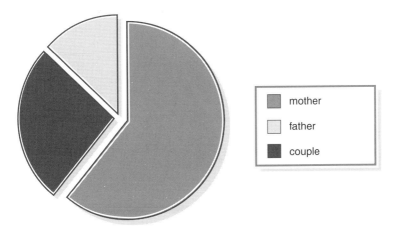

Figure 8.1   Interview sample by group (mother, father, couple).

Not all couples were married and some male interviewees were not the natural father of the child in PICU. When interviewed as a couple more data were obtained from the female partner. One disadvantage of interviewing after discharge from the PICU was that after the 'PICU crisis' many fathers either

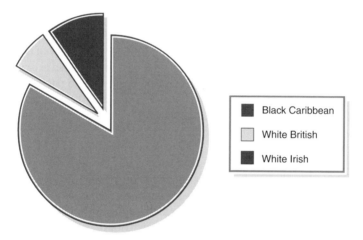

Black Caribbean

White British

White Irish

Figure 8.2   Ethnic origins of participants.

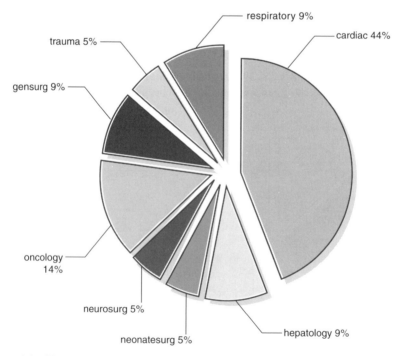

respiratory 9%

cardiac 44%

trauma 5%

gensurg 9%

oncology
14%

neurosurg 5%

neonatesurg 5%

hepatology 9%

Figure 8.3   Diagnostic codes of children of parents interviewed.

returned to work or went home to care for their other children, and were therefore unavailable for interview.

Ethnic origin is indicated in Figure 8.2. All non-English speaking parents were approached by a nurse who spoke their language. However, attempts to interview parents of Asian origin were unsuccessful. Explanations for the failure to recruit this ethnic group appear complex. In accordance with ethics guidelines families were not asked to give a reason why they did not wish to participate, although some parents volunteered information. The main reason for refusal to participate appeared to be that parents did not wish to leave their child's bedside while they were in hospital, or were attending to extended family at home. Refusal to participate was either stated explicitly, or demonstrated by non-attendance for interview at arranged times.

Sampling was convenience in nature and a breakdown of diagnosis is illustrated in Figure 8.3, although the sample is fairly representative of the population of children cared for in PICU.

Length of stay of children is illustrated in Figure 8.4. It ranged from 0.8 to 21.5 PICU days.

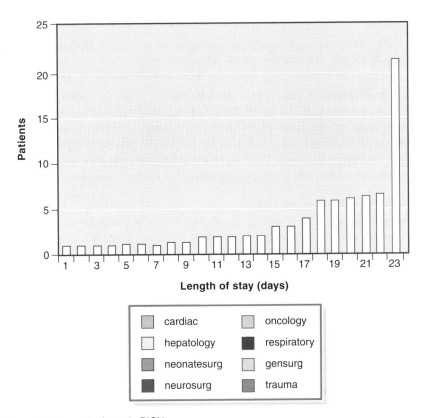

Figure 8.4 Length of stay in PICU.

Themes identified

Interviews were transcribed and the data examined for the occurrence of common themes. The themes identified were not dissimilar to those identified in previous research, which further validates this study. However, the phenomenological approach yielded rich data and identified areas for further study.

Stress and distress

Given the nature of the PICU it was not surprising that there was an overwhelming theme of stress and distress for parents of critically ill children. This appeared less so for planned admissions, but it should not be forgotten that even for parents who have had extensive preoperative admission and support, the first sight of their child in the PICU can be overwhelming.

There was nothing that we didn't expect, but of course if it's your own child it's heart wrenching. It wasn't a shock; the fact that she was lying there peacefully made it easier. But your heart goes out, all your worries come flooding back.

Mother (Child planned cardiac admission)

… really shocked. Even though we had all the information, it doesn't really sink in until you see your child.

Mother (Child planned cardiac admission)

The first thing I thought was this is a bit intimidating. When you first actually go in you see this huge space with a lot people working in different uniforms.

Father (Child oncology emergency admission)

A number of parents were not prepared for the open plan unit and were distressed at seeing other children. They had expected the unit to be divided into cubicles. Parents who visited PICU prior to their child's admission, however, preferred the openness of the unit and said the relaxed attitude of many PICU staff helped to lessen their stress. They also felt that junior nurses were always able to summon assistance from senior colleagues and found that reassuring.

Readiness to receive information

Parents of cardiac patients usually undergo an extensive preoperative information programme, including a visit to PICU. Parents referred to getting all the information they needed from the nurses and doctors. However, there were some issues that arose as a result of discussion with parents that require further exploration:

* When did parents feel really ready to receive the information?
* Are short repetitive bursts better or in one big block followed by specific, short directive blocks?
* Do parents need more written information (or less, as this might heighten stress in the PICU situation)?
* Who should give them the information? Is there a clear communication pathway where parents know who to get information from (building on named nurse, etc.) or is it ad hoc?

- Skills and experience of nurses delivering/giving information?
- How do others know what has been said? Specific documentation or not?

Parents of children who were admitted for planned procedures appeared better informed than those who were emergency admissions. Parents of emergency admissions to PICU will not always be receptive to information. This is taken into consideration in communicating with parents in PICU. A communication sheet is included in the nursing documentation and includes any information relayed to parents.

Furthermore, the amount of information parents are able to retain when they are distressed about their child's condition should not be overestimated, as illustrated by the response of a mother who was asked if she was given any information prior to seeing her child on the PICU:

I couldn't honestly remember, I'm not sure that I would remember if I did.

Mother (Child emergency admission)

In reference to the amount of information given following admission to the PICU, parents felt that procedures were explained mainly by nursing staff:

… Nobody ever did anything without explaining first.

Mother (Child emergency admission)

When asked what she thought 'intensive care' meant, one mother expressed the following opinion:

I thought it was the last stop, I thought he was going to die.

Mother (Child emergency admission)

This demonstrates the preconceived ideas some parents may have about the PICU. Parents of planned cardiac admissions viewed PICU as a necessary part of their child's care, and although pleased to leave PICU, were mainly positive about their experience there. Having being admitted with her child over ten years previously, one mother made comparisons between the information given now and previously.

Things have moved on so much on the ward and ICU. They communicate more. When—had his first op we only saw him (the surgeon) once. The surgeon this time was wonderful he didn't make us feel like he was a doctor. He was very approachable. They seem to talk to the parents and child much more informally. They make sure you understand and if you don't, then they tell you to ask.

Mother (Child planned admission)

We were very clear. We were told that however silly a question might seem, always ask and the nurse will make time to answer. That was a good point, that stood you in good stead. So when you were in intensive care you remembered that and weren't afraid to ask.

Father (Child emergency admission)

Being with their child and knowing and trusting the PICU staff

Parents described how they trusted the PICU staff. Parents of long-stay children described how they came to think of the nurses as friends:

They don't come across as doctors and nurses to me – they are people that care.

Mother (Child emergency admission)

Many parents spoke of forming friendships with the PICU staff. Some staff were singled-out as doing 'more than their job':

She's one of these people I could walk out of here and say 'Give us your telephone number, I'd like to keep in touch with you' because she really took care of—and us, especially me.

Mother (Child emergency admission)

Knowing and trusting the PICU nurses meant that parents were able to go for breaks while their child was in the PICU:

I was really surprised that there was one nurse to every bed so I used that opportunity to get a break for myself because I felt—was really safe.

Mother (Child planned admission)

However, one parent described how she did not trust one nurse:

For the two 6 hour shifts that this particular nurse worked I couldn't go. I even got my Mum to come up for the 2 hours that we went home. I just hadn't got any confidence in her whatsoever.

Not surprisingly some parents would not leave their child in PICU, even for short periods of time. Understandably, as well as trusting the staff, this appears to be related to how unstable parents perceived their child to be:

… I would never forgive myself if something happened and I wasn't there. I know its not going to happen in minutes, cause I knew he was on a ventilator, but I couldn't forgive myself if I hadn't been there at the time.

Mother (Child emergency admission)

Vicarious grieving and guilt

As mentioned previously, the PICU is spacious and mainly open-plan in design, along with cubicles and more private areas. Some parents commented on the lack of privacy during times of distress. When the unit is full there may be more than 40 parents around at any one time. Many parents viewed the parents' room as spacious. However, a number of parents said that the room was not big enough and the provision of a 'happy room' and a 'quiet room' would be a good idea:

… personal space for people to grieve. When we cracked up we were in a cubicle so when we were shouting 'come on—don't give up now' we couldn't be heard, but, there was one distraught mother in the parents' room and I had to come out … because it was too close to home … to listen to someone who was going through the same thing we were going through and obviously being a day behind us.

Mother (Child emergency admission)

Parents also related how they became friends with other parents on the unit and the feelings of guilt they experienced when their child was doing well and others were detoriating.

Transfer to the ward
This study was concerned with the period children and parents were on PICU; however, some parents offered information about their stay on the wards. Parents of planned short-stay admissions viewed going to the ward as a sign that their child was recovering. However, parents of emergency admissions spoke of their shock and apprehension when transfer to the ward was mentioned. Transfer to the ward was not always felt to be discussed early enough. Additionally, some parents felt that there was a lack of appreciation by ward staff of what they had been through on PICU.

Specific issues raised by fathers
There were a number of issues raised by fathers which were largely of a security and managerial nature. This was an interesting finding, as many of the mothers focused on care, relationship and communication issues. One of the fathers highlighted concern about nurses working long shifts and not having breaks. Another mentioned the need for better directions to the hospital.

Discussion
The majority of interviews were carried out with mothers. One possible explanation for this was the absence of fathers from the hospital, particularly when the life-threatening phase of their child's illness was seen to be over. Many fathers returned to work or went home to care for siblings. It was also clear that many women viewed their partner as being less able to cope with their child's intensive care stay. These gender differences require further exploration.

Attempts to interview parents whose first language was not English were unsuccessful; this was despite originally having a nurse specialist who spoke Asian languages on the team. It would have been unethical to ask families to give reasons why they did not want to be involved in the study, although it further serves to highlight the cultural differences present, a topic which requires investigation. One family volunteered information that the cultural difference meant that the extended family were often cared for by the parent that was not at the hospital. A multi-professional study is currently being planned, where non-English speaking families will be surveyed. In addition the patient/family journey of the child who stays in PICU long term requires further research.

Implications for practice
As a result of this study parental involvement in the planning of PICU services at BCH Trust now includes the following:

- All parents of children admitted to PICU should be offered a questionnaire consisting of a number of open/closed questions.

- Parents of long-stay PICU children should be invited back for interviews. (There is an existing PICU bereavement support programme.)
- The possibility of parent forums should be explored.

SUMMARY AND CONCLUSION

This chapter has outlined the development of a research database and drawn on some examples from practice made available to the wider nursing community in one children's hospital as a result of that source of information.

The aim of presenting the exemplars in this chapter was to highlight some of clinical research undertaken by children's nurses. The PRAM database helped to bring such projects to the awareness of others, both within the trust and further afield. As the PRAM project has grown and evolved, the trust now has a formal network of nursing research activities mapped in a user-friendly database. Through its joint leadership it has provided a unique opportunity for children's nurses at the trust to link together under the umbrella of research. Indeed, the PRAM group has come a long way since the initiation and arguably has the potential to go even further.

The research framework was used to help underpin the process of change and as a result research skills have been developed within the group. In the future it is intended that, through this database, potential research projects, including multidisciplinary work, will be identified. Furthermore, the joint participation between the university and clinical areas of the trust has served to facilitate the linking of theory to practice. This has meant that lecturing staff in education and clinical staff in the hospital trust can be rallied to generate additional interest and support for the project.

It is hoped that the contents of this chapter have illustrated, inspired and motivated nurses to embark on a journey that will contribute to the advancement of child health and indeed nursing. It is hoped that this will add to the body of evidence-based nursing to take it forward into a new dimension.

REFERENCES

Abbott K 1990 Therapeutic use of play in the psychological preparation of pre-school children undergoing cardiac surgery. Pediatric Nursing 13(4): 265–277
Boatwright D N, Crummette B D 1991 Preparing children for endoscopy and manometry. Gastroenterology Nursing 13(3): 142–145
Boliq R, Yolton K A, Nissen H L 1991 Medical care and preparation, questions and issues. Children Healthcare 20(4): 225–229
Bradshaw P L 1995 The recent health reforms in the United Kingdom: some tentative observations on their impact on nurses and nursing in hospitals. Journal of Advanced Nursing 21(5): 975–979

Callery P 1997 Caring for parents of hospitalised children: a hidden area of nurse's work. Journal of Advanced Nursing 26: 992–998

Collaizi P 1978 Psychological research as a phenomenologist views it. In: Existential phenomenological alternatives for psychology. Valle R, King M (eds) Oxford University Press, New York

Coad J et al 2001 The development of research through a nursing database at a regional children's hospital. Paediatric Nursing 13(9): November

Department of Health 1997a Paediatric intensive care 'A framework for the future': National Coordinating Group on Paediatric Intensive Care. Report to the Chief Executive of the NHS Executive. HMSO, London

Department of Health 1997b A bridge to the future: nursing standards, education and workforce planning in paediatric intensive care. Report of the Chief Nursing Officers Taskforce. HMSO, London

Department of Health 2000 The NHS plan. HMSO, London

Department of Health 2003 Emerging findings (national service framework for children, young people and maternity services). April. DoH, London

Ellerton M L, Ritchie J S, Caty S 1994 Factors influencing young children's coping behaviours during stressful healthcare encounters. Maternal Child Nursing Journal 22(3): 74–82

Farrel M F, Frost C 1992 The most important needs of parents of critically ill children: parents perceptions. Intensive and Critical Care Nursing 8(3): 130–139

Fisher M D 1994 Identified needs of parents in a pediatric intensive care unit. Critical Care Nurse 14(3): 82–90

Funk S, Champagne M, Wiese R, Tournquist E 1991 Barriers: the barriers to research utilisation scale. Applied Nursing Research 4: 39–45

Glasper A, Venn C, Roberts A 1992 Preparing for hospital. Cascade 6: 3–4

Higher Education Funding Council for England 2001 Research in nursing and allied health professions: Report of Task Group 3. Hefce and Department of Health, London

Holden C, MacDonald A 2000 (eds) Nutrition and child health. Baillière Tindall, Edinburgh

Holden C E, MacDonald A, Ward M et al 1997 Psychological preparation for nasogastric feeding in children. British Journal of Nursing 6(7): 376–385

Hunsberger M, Love B, Byrne C 1994 A review of current approaches used to help children and parents cope with healthcare procedures. Maternal Child Nursing Journal 13(3): 145–165

Jay S M 1988 Invasive medical procedures: psychological intervention and assessment. In: Routh D K (ed) Handbook of pediatric psychology. Guildford Press, New York: 401–425

Lee R M 1993 Doing research on sensitive topics. Sage Publications, London

Mansson M E, Fredrikzon B, Rosberg B 1992 Comparison of preparation and narcotic-sedative pre-medication in children undergoing surgery. Paediatric Nursing 18(4): 337–342, 350–351

Melamed B G, Ridley-Johnson R 1988 Psychological preparation of families for hospitalisation. Developments in Behavioural Pediatrics 9: 96–102

Molter N 1979 Needs of relatives of critically ill patients: a descriptive study. Heart and Lung 8: 332–339

Noyes J 1998 A critique of studies exploring the experiences and needs of parents of children admitted to paediatric intensive care. Journal of Advanced Nursing 28(1): 134–141

Rope R N, Bush J P 1994 Psychological preparation for pediatric oncology patients undergoing painful procedures: a methodological critique of research. Children Healthcare 23(1): 51–67

Vessey J A, Carlson K L, McGill J 1994 Use of distraction with children during an acute pain experience. Nursing Research 43(6): 369–372

Walsh M 1997 How nurses perceive barriers to research implementation. Nursing Standard 11(29): 34–39

Young M H 1994 Preparation for nasogastric tube placement: psychological support. In: Baker S B, Baker R D, Davis A (eds) Paediatric enteral nutrition. Chapman and Hall, London

9

Experiences in mental health nursing

Maureen Smojkis   Peter Nolan

Editors' comment

This chapter offers a comprehensive overview of the challenges of developing a research agenda in one branch of nursing, namely mental health. The challenges of doing so in this specialist field of practice are well illustrated and the examples of experience of working to change the agenda emphasize some of the points raised in earlier chapters about managing organizational change. This is complemented by a focused project in primary care in which researchers' experience of an action research approach is outlined.

INTRODUCTION

Until relatively recently, the theory and practice of mental health nursing have been largely driven by a top-down approach. A variety of influences including mental health commissioners, service providers, doctors, psychologists, healthcare policies and practice guidelines have been far more important in defining the work of the mental health nurse than any findings resulting from research into mental health nursing. A brief overview of the evolution of research into mental health nursing may provide some explanation for this state of affairs while demonstrating that mental health nursing in the past did not constitute a robust body of knowledge contributed to by a sophisticated group of professionals.

Although training for mental health nurses in the UK was first introduced in 1891 and the scheme was the first national scheme of its kind anywhere in the world, it took several decades before all mental health care institutions were participating in it. This was because, at the end of the 19th century, there was great variation between psychiatrists and hospital administrators as to what constituted effective treatment for mental illness and, indeed, what the overall aims of mental health services were. The constant finding in mental health services since their inception in the mid-19th century was that they experienced considerable difficulties in recruiting high quality personnel willing and able to form a critical mass to improve care and generate a theoretical basis for best practice. The optimism that accompanied the incorporation of mental health services into the NHS in 1948 was short-lived for it was found that there was no intention to integrate mental health care with mainstream acute services. In fact, the reverse was the case, as the separation from other healthcare services was exacerbated by the provision of pathological laboratories, radiology facilities, pharmacies and research departments within the mental hospitals themselves, rendering any communication with general health services unnecessary. Only a few Medical Research Council (MRC) funded psychiatric research departments were created in the early days of the NHS and these were beginning to fade out by the mid-1970s. Their contribution to raising the quality of care provided to the majority of people with mental health problems in the UK was highly questionable. Though only a few nurses were employed in these units, their role was mainly confined to collecting specimens from patients and conveying them to the laboratories for analysis. These units were predominantly medically dominated and they were characterized by a search for long-lasting treatments as opposed to finding ways of improving care and support for people with mental health problems.

The newly formed NHS was principally concerned with the management of acute hospitals and it was there that most of its resources were targeted. It was almost a decade before attention turned to psychiatric hospitals when it became apparent that almost three-quarters of the beds provided by the NHS were occupied by patients with a multitude of psychiatric illnesses. Those whose responsibility it was to keep NHS costs within affordable limits could consult no substantial body of research into the management and care of patients with mental health problems. Only the MRC units were undertaking any research in psychiatry during the 1950s and their focus was not on examining the social climate of hospitals or the therapeutic benefits they provided for patients. Issues of this kind were addressed inconsistently and on an irregular basis by periodic internal inquiries carried out by administrators.

THE BEGINNINGS OF MENTAL HEALTH NURSING RESEARCH

The first serious attempts to explore the work of mental nurses, although not undertaken by nurses, were made by the Liverpool Regional Hospital Board (1954), by Oppenheim & Ereman (1955) and by the Manchester Regional Hospital Board (1956). These were followed by two studies designed and undertaken by nurses (Maddox 1957, John 1961). It is not coincidental that these studies were undertaken at a time when healthcare costs were escalating at an alarming rate and Ministry of Health officials were expressing concern that they could not be sustained. All the studies concluded that mental nursing was difficult to define and that only some aspects of the nurse's work had any claim to be related to patient care. The Liverpool study identified serious staff shortages and noted that while in 1938 there had been 194 student nurses in training, that number had fallen to 28 by

1953. Between 1948 and 1953, over two-thirds of those who commenced training dropped out. The twin problems of maintaining staffing levels and attempting to provide some degree of training for those who stayed presented a lamentable picture of mental health nursing at that time. The Manchester study, in particular, concluded that most of the work of nurses was not especially skilled and could be conducted by untrained assistants, although in a later study Gallagher et al (1957) warned against the wide-scale employment of nursing assistants. These nurses, the study argued, tended to adopt authoritarian roles, distanced themselves from patients and tended to see their remit solely as enforcing order within the organization. Only nursing assistants staffed many wards in some hospitals and they ignored or avoided whatever was deemed to be good practice at the time.

These studies suggested that the culture of the Poor Law on which the asylums had been founded and run for many decades was still flourishing in the 1950s. It was not until a series of very public inquiries was held in the 1960s and 1970s that the extent of the entrenched nature of attitudes and practices in psychiatric hospitals was revealed (Martin 1984). Ignoring the high levels of neglect that prevailed within mental hospitals could no longer be sustained. Eighteen public inquiries and many private ones highlighted the inadequacies of the system of mental health care, the deplorable state of mental health care provided by nurses, and the appalling lack of concern and vision on the part of those entrusted with the management of hospitals. These revelations of the inadequacies in mental health care brought to the fore the first mental health nurses with a background and training in research. First and foremost among these was Annie Altschul (1972), the UK's first professor of psychiatric nursing, at Edinburgh University. Altschul was fully aware that without an inquiring, curious and informed nursing workforce the work had no direction and many nurses perceived their contribution to patient care to be, at best, of little consequence. She set about creating a theoretical basis for nursing and challenged nurses to understand what nursing was and how it worked (Barker 1999, 2002). She was one of the first British mental health nurses to undertake a prolonged educational visit to the USA to observe at first hand and learn from a number of eminent American nurses including Hildegard Peplau. On her return to the UK, Altschul saw that factors such as social isolation, alienation and anomie played a large part in causing the mental illnesses of patients admitted to the Maudsley Hospital in London. What these patients needed above all, she considered, were human relationships, preferably with educated, compassionate nurses. Hence, her first writings were devoted to nurse–patient relationships. She saw nurses as ideally placed to assist patients in rediscovering their abilities to make and sustain relationships. While other professionals specialized in meeting other particular needs, whether these were biomedical, social or financial, nurses should seek to encompass the whole person. She stressed the importance of the therapeutic relationship in mental health nursing and this has been the one activity most significantly noted by users of the mental health services to date.

Other researchers influenced by Altschul's work included Towell (1975), Cormack (1976), Clinton (1981) and Pollock (1982). Though all of them drew attention to the importance of researching mental health nursing they continued to find little of therapeutic value in what nurses did; most of the work of mental health nurses consisted of low-level administrative tasks and acting as servants to doctors. Nurse education was found to be perpetuating the ethos of the institutions, impressing on students the importance of following rules, being doctor dependent and deferring all decisions to senior personnel. Such training inevitably turned out nurses who were only able to function within traditional institutions, who saw care as being the imposition of routines and restricted behaviours and who were quite unable to challenge the status quo or be innovative in their thinking or practice.

THE SEARCH FOR A NEW DIRECTION

In order to address the revelations made by the public inquiries of mistreatment of patients in some psychiatric hospitals, the Nodder Report (DHSS 1979) suggested that links between psychiatric services and general practitioners (GPs) should be enhanced. Hospital-based nursing staff were to be trained in change management, and specialist training for community psychiatric nurses (CPNs) was to commence in keeping with plans to close the large institutions and expand community care (Gournay & Beardsmoore 1995). They also argued that quality assurance in mental health nursing could best be achieved by ensuring that those who wrote the standards would be those who implemented them. This initiative was nurse led but, unlike the *Essence of Care, Benchmarking* (Department of Health 2001), did not focus on the inclusion of clients.

In 1992, a major review of mental health nursing in the UK was commenced. It received evidence concerning the enormous changes in social structures and family life in the UK over the previous three decades, the increased need for child protection and the lack of representation of women and ethnic minority groups in the mental health services (Owen 2001). It was put to the review body that mental health nursing at all levels must embrace the use of outcome measures and that assessment and evaluation should be directed by expert nurse researchers (Gallop 1998).

Working in Partnership (Department of Health 1993) expanded on these recommendations, insisting that mental health nurses must be accountable for the standards of care they provide in order to meet the challenge of developing high-quality mental health nursing services. The core skills of the mental health nurse were defined in terms of interpersonal relationships and operational flexibility. The report rejected the creation of a 'generic' nurse or the conversion of mental health nursing to a post-registration speciality and recommended that urgent and committed attention be given to developing research skills among mental health nurses through funded support from management. Nurses would then be able to identify what should be the essential work of mental health nurses, and who were their natural clients.

Nolan (1995), among others, further highlighted the lack of a unique philosophy of mental health nursing to structure its practices. Other recent researchers have tried to develop such a philosophy. For instance Barker et al (1999) spent five years exploring what people 'need psychiatric nurses for' and concluded that 'sometimes people need someone to take care of them, and at other times they need someone to take with them' and that this fits with 'person-centred' care in its broadest sense. Barker's tidal model (Barker 2001) extends and develops some of the traditional assumptions concerning the centrality of interpersonal relations in nursing practice and is clearly influenced by the work of Altschul and Peplau. Barker suggests that the time is ripe for nurses to explore new ways of caring *with* people (while continuing to care for and about them) and of facilitating an understanding of such a process in the people who are in their care. Graham (2001) sought to understand the craft of mental health nursing in terms of the practice of a community mental health team in the UK. The team felt that mental health nursing was characterized by holism, relationship building, partnership and empowerment.

Research into mental health nursing is still in its infancy despite the fact that *Psychiatric Nursing Today and Tomorrow* (1968) predicted a substantial growth in research undertaken by British mental health nurses. Dodd (2001) suggests that mental health care has struggled with the notion of translating research into practice ever since it began to focus on treatment rather than segregation. Despite being part of the nursing agenda for the last 30 years, the notion of research continues to cause anxiety for many nurses. This anxiety seems to be founded on an idea that clinical work and research activity are separate activities, a feeling that nurses are the subject of research rather than the instigator, and the notion that evidence-based practice is delivered to, rather than influenced by, the practitioner. Such attitudes highlight the need for the integration of research into the delivery of mental health care from the beginning of the nurse's career, in the pre-registration or undergraduate arena, and its continuation through professional development.

Barker (1999) argued that all psychiatric nurses need to become 'research literate', either through formal academic exercises or by engaging in practical, hands-on studies. Cheek (2000) insists that research into aspects of nursing is an activity which should be predominantly the concern of nurses.

CURRENT FOCUS OF RESEARCH IN MENTAL HEALTH NURSING

An examination of the literature shows the diversity of research that has been carried out in the field of psychiatric/mental health nursing on a national and international level. Researchers include academics, clinicians, service users and other disciplines working either independently or in collaborative ventures. In a review of US nursing literature from 1989 to 1994 Merwin & Mauck (1995) found that few psychiatric nursing studies were published in major research journals and that few studies built on prior research, thus failing to contribute to the establishment of a strong research basis for evaluating the outcomes of psychiatric nursing care. However, the authors admit to being selective in their choice of articles for review and to having omitted many that focused on the psychosocial needs of clients with various physical conditions.

Over the past 50 years in the UK, the focus of mental health research has shifted from an activity that was predominantly conducted outside the clinical arena to a collaborative undertaking focused on and in the clinical process and how it impacts on service user and carer. Table 9.1 illustrates this change in focus and process.

Schon (1983), Burnard & Hannigan (2000) and Burnard (2002) propose that the research agenda is dictated by two opposing parties: (1) quantitative researchers who argue in favour of experimental research which investigates the outcomes of nursing care, is multidisciplinary, favours physiological explanations for mental illness, and supports evidence-based practice and skills-based education, and (2) qualitative researchers who explore the *experience* of illness and of nursing, are advocates of nursing research conducted by nurses alone, find physiological explanations of mental illness irrelevant, and support a holistic approach to mental health nursing where interpersonal relationships rather than techniques are

Table 9.1 Changing focus of nursing research

Period	Research emphasis
Pre 1960	Researcher as expert Research generated in response to concerns about public safety Researcher as crusader
1980s and 1990s	Research directed by Department of Health Priority areas identified Tendering by individuals for research monies
2000s	Service users and carers seen to be central to the research agenda Collaboration in research between disciplines Collaboration between researchers and providers of services Collaboration with education sector Research in the clinical arena

paramount. However, Burnard & Hannigan (2000) conclude that the two approaches are different in emphasis rather than in fundamentals.

The influence of logical positivism has been strong in healthcare research and has influenced both its subject matter and the research methods employed. Cheek (2000), however, argues that there is room for all kinds of methodologies in nursing and, indeed, that it should not commit itself to any one methodology in particular. What is required is the recognition by nurses that research is one of the profession's core functions, and a growing awareness of how research findings can assist nurses to grapple with the demands of an increasingly diverse and complex professional role.

Current focus: acute in-patient services

Over the past 5 years, the provision of mental health care in acute in-patient settings has become a key area for research. The reconfiguration of mental health care involving the closure of the large institutions and the reduction in the number of beds has impacted in ways that were not predicted. The Mental Health Act Commission (1997) identified a shortfall in resources in acute settings with serious implications for care provision. The morale of mental health nurses working in these settings has fallen as the attention of policy makers and providers has increasingly shifted to nurses providing care in the community. Education and professional development opportunities have proliferated for community nurses since the early 1990s (e.g. the Thorn initiative which emphasized the importance of psychosocial interventions with families, and the Birmingham community mental health course), while there are no such courses for post-registration nurses working in in-patient settings. Hence the Sainsbury Centre for Mental Health (2001) remarked that acute in-patient wards across England are poorly supported educationally.

Barker (2000) identified that the focus in academic research on CPNs has inhibited the development of skills to carry out psychosocial care for people in acute psychiatric wards. The move towards crisis management which has contributed to a reduction in patient contact time has also increased nurses' stress levels. Barker suggests that strategies for tackling such problems in acute in-patient settings might include: assessment by the team of its priorities; supernumerary status of staff in order to be able to carry out assessment of clients; specific interventions, and improved time management and planning. Dodd & Wellman (2000) have added to the literature by examining how staff development programmes in acute psychiatric in-patient settings, and training in anxiety and relaxation techniques, for both staff and patients, are both possible and effective.

Dodds & Bowles (2001) reported on the reorganization of patient care on an inner-city acute 21-bedded in-patient ward for males under the age of 65. The team acted on reports from previous literature and reorganized patient care and nursing care without formal observation. The report showed how the use of a structured programme, change to formal observation policy and nursing practice showed, over a 6-month period, a reduction in formal observation and an increase in structured individualized activity. The study identified a reduction in the incidence of deliberate self-harm, violence and absconding and a reduction in length of stay, staff sickness and staffing costs.

Taylor et al (2002) report on the findings of a practice development study aiming to improve the quality of small group work within an in-patient facility. The four ward teams adopted a modified version of Irvin Yalom's higher-level model of in-patient group therapy and ran thrice weekly 1-hour sessions. Using quantitative and qualitative methods, the researchers found that rather than improving practice, a decline in quality became apparent during the 6-month period of the study. This they attributed to the increase in the ward team's workload caused by the sessions; inadequate staffing levels; and changes in expectations of those providing the small group therapy. Taylor et al (2002) commented that the failure of the project raises questions about the effectiveness of action learning as a developmental method. In their opinion, action learning (see Ch. 4) is most likely to be effective when participants focus on practice that lies directly within their control and that attempts to use it as a vehicle for pursuing change on a wider front are likely to fail. This study provides an excellent example of the way in which research can assist and reflect on the development of practice.

Current focus: medication management

Mental health in primary care and medication management are now emerging as key issues for research in the UK. Interest in nurse prescribing has increased within the past 10 years. The *NHS Plan* (Department of Health 2000) states that the majority of nurses will be able to prescribe by the year 2004. For mental health nurses, this means an extension of their traditional role of administering medication and observing for side-effects. The importance of this part of the mental health nurse's role has been the subject of considerable debate. Gournay & Beardsmoore (1995) found that CPNs and Thorn graduates saw medication interventions as an important part of their role, with both groups stating that they asked patients at least once a month about the side-effects of anti-psychotic drugs. However, assessment tools were used more frequently by Thorn graduates than CPNs, who had not completed the programme.

The study carried out by Nolan et al (2001), which explored mental health nurses' perceptions of the advantages and disadvantages of nurse prescribing and asked them to identify the educational needs of mental health nurse prescribers, will assist in the development of mental health care in the coming years. Crawford et al's study (2001) examining the impact of community mental health nurses (CMHN) placed in two primary care practices is also relevant.

RESEARCH INTO PRACTICE

Getting research into practice is clearly a worthy aim that appears at first sight to be seductively simple. Few would seek actively to prevent the implementation of research-based interventions in order to improve the quality of care for people with mental health problems. For years, mental health professionals have been committed to grounding their practice in research and have achieved some degree of success. However, there have been obstacles. The National Institute for Mental Health in England was established in 2002 in order to respond firstly to the problem of research being undertaken idiosyncratically across the country, and secondly, to the issue of time lapse before the findings of high-quality research are taken up by practitioners. Much research appears never to find its way into anything other than the pages of journals or, even more regrettably, lies unpublished on the shelves of university academics. The National Institute aims to improve the quality of research, inform service providers about best practice in their area, help them incorporate research into existing practice, and assist policy makers in formulating realistic policies. It considers research to be a means of:

- Increasing job satisfaction and avoiding burnout
- Providing the best possible care for clients and their carers
- Involving clients in discovering how best to deliver services.

Perhaps more than any other group working in mental health care, mental health nurses feel especially challenged to become research aware. Their training and work are focused on service delivery; others engage in making clinical judgements, formulating care plans and taking overall responsibility for the management of clients. Since the 1970s and 1980s, people such as Davis (1986) have argued that mental health nurses must understand that nursing is not just about acquiring and demonstrating skills; it is also about extending skills and identifying new ones through undertaking and implementing research at all levels of the organization. The current profile of mental health nursing is heavily weighted towards engagement with clients and interpersonal problem-solving, while the skills of reading and critically analysing research and reflecting on and writing about practice are undervalued although equally important. It is now well established that for research to impact on the service setting, mental health nurses require skilled researchers who can collaborate and communicate with service colleagues, a workforce that is eager to accept and implement new ways of working, and management personnel who can create a favourable environment in which change can occur and be sustained.

Jorm (2000) reviewed a number of unsuccessful attempts to improve practice through research and identified various factors contributing to these failures. Firstly, he noted that the belief that the research project is complete once the final report has been written is common and fatal. Other difficulties include:

- Overambitious plans and time-scales
- Lack of organizational support
- An organization which accepts the need for change but does not have the infrastructure to deliver it
- An organization which accepts and delivers change, but fails to sustain it
- Over-dependence on a single charismatic leader
- Limited interagency endorsement
- Lack of long-term revenue planning.

RESEARCH INTO PRACTICE: THE AUTHORS' EXPERIENCE

In the mid 1990s, the authors set about seeking ways of getting research into practice in a large inner city mental health trust. The trust had a good reputation for encouraging nurses to attend courses on research, but it was not apparent what impact attendance was having on the nurses once they returned to their place of work – what innovations they instituted and with what success. Good relationships existed between one of the local universities and the trust's nursing department, and the authors, who worked at the university, invited mental health nurses with a known interest in research to a meeting to discuss how research findings could be incorporated into practice. It was decided to undertake a short survey among nurses to find the answers to the following questions:

- What education in research did they have?
- Had they carried out any research?
- What impact, if any, was their research having on their own practice or the practice of others?

In total, 350 questionnaires were distributed to a random sample of mental health nurses working in the trust. Unfortunately, only 14 (4%) were returned completed. These made it very clear that there was no coherent approach to training nurses in research. Respondents described their education in research as consisting of critiquing a paper, preparing a short literature review on a topic of their choice, or writing a short research proposal. None of the respondents had shared what they had learned with any colleagues, and the work they had undertaken had been seen only by their course tutors. Furthermore, it was implied in the responses that whatever research skills were acquired they were not regarded as having any relevance to where the nurses worked. Respondents reported that few people within the trust seemed to be interested in their studies or in research. These 14 completed questionnaires proved invaluable for the authors in establishing the baseline from which they would be working in their efforts to raise the level of research awareness among the nursing workforce.

Subsequently, members of the nursing department of the university and senior nurses from within the trust devised a strategy to get more nurses interested and involved in research. Stage 1 was to invite nurses who were attempting to incorporate research into practice in their service environments to three public seminars during 1996. The average attendance at each seminar was 150. Topics covered by the presenters included:

- Getting started in research
- Involving others in research
- Disseminating research findings within the organization
- Integrating research into job descriptions, agendas for meetings, supervision and individual appraisals.

Following these very successful seminars, it was decided to hold open-house meetings devoted to research issues on a monthly basis. A core group of eight people volunteered to arrange the meetings, set the agendas and take responsibility for maintaining the group. Rather to the organizers' surprise, doctors, occupational therapists and social workers were as keen to attend as mental health nurses. Many insights were gained from the discussions that took place at the early meetings, which were:

- Research requires time and resources if it is to be worthwhile, so has to be valued by the whole organization
- Interest in research cannot be imposed on nurses; it must be generated from within nursing – 'You cannot take nurses from where they are not to where they don't want to be!'
- Nurses should not feel under an obligation to do research.

Meetings and discussions took place on a regular basis for almost 2 years before it was decided to attempt to conduct the research that individuals wanted. Proposals were written and requests made to the trust for funding for three key projects:

1. Management of self-harming clients
2. Implementing the supervision register
3. Evaluating a liaison psychiatric service.

Within a few months, £50 000 had been generated, yet despite vigorous attempts to recruit nurses to combine a master's degree with taking the lead role in these projects, only one would commit herself for 18 months to the management of self-harming clients project. The other projects were eventually led by psychology graduates.

Each project leader was supervised by both a member of academic staff from the university and a senior clinical person with research experience from the trust. As time progressed, it became obvious that:

1. Supervision was more time-consuming than had been originally intended.
2. Although ethical permission had been sought and granted for all three projects, some staff refused to collaborate with the researchers, referring to them as 'strangers' and 'intruders'.
3. Several attempts to collect data were unsuccessful, despite arrangements having been made in advance, because emergencies arose and there were staff shortages.
4. There were problems in locating offices for the project leads, in getting computers for them, and in finding expertise to help them analyse their data.

It also became apparent that the nurse lead was highly motivated and was having a considerable impact on her service colleagues, while the two psychology leads lacked confidence. They did not understand the NHS culture or the differences between professional groups. They were therefore uncertain how to feed information back to staff in order to raise research awareness. It seemed that a nurse with a sound knowledge of research and leadership skills was the best person to assist the process of getting research into practice, to collaborate with nurses in particular settings and keep them informed. Nurses were prepared to change their behaviour, rewrite procedures and guidelines and implement them in practice when the person charged with getting research into practice was actively engaged with nursing colleagues (see Ch. 4). On the other hand, where there was little involvement of the project leads with nurses, outcomes were disappointing.

The core group had been taken aback by the reluctance of nurses to put themselves forward for the research posts and began to consider the possibility of linking research training to clinical work via a multidisciplinary postgraduate master's course in health sciences. The course included modules in health service policy and management, change theory, health economics and research methods, and required students to carry out a piece of research related to their clinical area. The core group circulated information about the master's degree to all nurses in the trust, inviting those interested to write a short research proposal. Study time was guaranteed, as was full payment of course fees, a book allowance, funding for conferences and access to computer facilities. Three studentships were subsequently awarded to nurses clearly committed to improving patient care in their clinical areas and who had the support of their managers. In the following 2 years, five further studentships were awarded.

The small number of applications for studentships provided further evidence to the core group that nurses lacked enthusiasm for research and confidence in their ability to do it. Many nurses who were interested in the studentships were anxious that they did not have the appropriate skills, and that a master's course would be beyond their abilities. It was apparent that raising research awareness and increasing nurses' willingness to undertake research would entail a considerable effort.

The nurses who received the first studentships did indeed find the academic level of the course demanding. Nonetheless, all were successful in obtaining their master's degree and made an excellent contribution to patient care by sharing their knowledge and skills with other members of their multidisciplinary teams. They arranged placements for themselves in different clinical areas to broaden their understanding of different approaches to care and initiated weekly meetings and journal clubs where staff could discuss best practice. Managers came to see them as a useful resource and consulted them about improving services and creating new ones. The impact made by the students was ultimately out of all proportion to their numbers. As they progressed through their master's courses, other members of staff who wanted to advance their own professional development increasingly approached the core group members.

PROFESSIONAL DEVELOPMENT INITIATIVE

Another key development was a joint professional development initiative between the nursing division at the university and clinical practice. This involved working with a primary care liaison team that is organized around the functionalized community mental service model, upon which the *National Service Framework (NSF) for Mental Health* (Department of Health 1999a) is largely based. The project was to introduce the team to solution-focused therapy (SFT), implement and evaluate the use of the interventions in practice.

The team

The primary care liaison team is a busy community mental health team, integrating health and social services. It is based in an inner-city area of 60 000 people making up a diverse socioeconomic and cultural population, with high psychiatric morbidity. The team has five key tasks:

1. Liaison with primary care services
2. Initial screening and assessment of clients with mental health problems
3. To be a single point of contact with psychiatric services
4. Casework with clients, most of whom would meet the criteria for the enhanced care programme approach (CPA) (Department of Health 1991)
5. To provide psychological therapies.

Clients access the team via primary care and are assessed and referred on to appropriate services. Clients and carers can receive a range of therapeutic interventions in line with the mental health NSF (Department of Health 1999a). The team comprises 25 staff from a variety of cultural and ethnic backgrounds and includes administrative assistants. The majority of clinical personnel are from nursing backgrounds. It was clear from the start that a multi-professional approach to professional development was essential in this team, although initially, the focus was on the nurses' needs in relation to PREP and *Making a Difference* (Department of Health 1999b) with the emphasis on lifelong learning.

Solution-focused therapy

Health services, by their nature, have been established in a problem-focused tradition, and mental health services are no exception. Research indicates that solution-focused interventions (SFIs) are of value in the mental health arena (Wilgosh et al 1992, Bowles 2001). The aim is to stay as close to the client's agenda as possible, and to find out what works for them by developing a strong collaborative relationship and a clear picture of the client's goals (O'Connell 1998).

One of the central assumptions is that the individual and the people around him or her may already possess the solutions to the issues which are causing *dis-ease*, and the interactions between the client and the worker involve assisting the client to rediscover these solutions through the narrative process. Wales (1998) believes that solution-focused therapy (SFT) can offer mental health nurses a robust framework on which to build appropriate and effective nursing interventions.

The project

At the beginning of this project a meeting was held with clinical staff to determine what aspects of their practice they felt needed to be developed. An agreement was reached that they would like to improve their approaches to therapy, and SFI was seen as one means of doing this. It was agreed that use of this approach would be introduced in a structured way and that the processes would be monitored and evaluated so that impact on service could be clearly reported.

An introductory workshop was arranged to introduce SFIs to members of the team who had stated an interest. Making links with the mental health arena, the team examined the assumptions of the model:

- Clients have the resources to make changes
- Clients define the goal
- There are always exceptions to problems (see below)
- Successful work depends on knowing where the client wants to get to
- Sometimes only the smallest of changes is necessary to set in motion a solution to the problem

- It is the task of the mental health worker to discover the best way to work alongside the client.

Four specifics of SFT were identified as being of particular value for the team:

Problem-free talk The worker is encouraged to connect with the person of the client and to begin to identify in conversation the skills, resources and strengths that the client has used in the past and that may be useful in the present.

Goal setting If clearly defined goals are not set, the client and worker will not be able to establish that progress is being made towards them or when they have been achieved.

Exception finding In relation to every problem, there are times when it is less worrying. Identifying such times can be the beginning of the process of reducing the power the problem has over the client's life. The worker needs to ask: 'What are you doing differently and what are others doing that is different at these (exceptional) times?'

Scaling questions Scaling questions can be used to measure change and thereby empower the client with a sense that he or she is moving forward and taking control. Such a question might be: 'On a scale of 1 to 10, with 1 being the worst that things have been around the issue and 10 representing how you want things to be, where are you today?' With further exploration, the worker can assist clients to identify what will be different when they have achieved movement towards the top of the scale, and boost their confidence that they can reach it.

The team also discussed how SFIs are likely to be more successful if approaches that the client has found useful in the past are identified. Appropriate questions might be:

- When you faced this sort of issue in the past, how did you resolve it?
- How could you do that again?
- What would need to happen for you to do that again?
- What other situations like this have you handled?

Following this, an open group took place every fortnight to offer support with the integration of SFI into clinical practice; this was facilitated by one of the authors who is a university-based lecturer and works clinically using an SFI approach. An established lecturer practitioner who uses SFTs with individuals and families also provided training and consultation.

The evaluation was undertaken using focus groups that explored the positive and negative aspects of using this approach and identified lessons that could be used to further develop practice. Common difficulties were identified. These included feelings of 'being stuck' with clients with whom staff had been in contact for some time; lack of shared understanding of issues between the client and the mental health worker; difficulty establishing that the purpose of the contact was different from that of other disciplines within the team. Positive aspects included the emergence of closer multi-professional working and the opportunity to share concerns and anxieties in using this approach to work. The groups recommended that there was a need to provide ongoing support and supervision in relation to SFI. This was provided by the lecturer practitioner. The support was provided as requested, for example two further study days were held for team members and clinical supervision sessions were maintained as required over a period of several months.

Summary of project

1. Identification of practice development need
2. Identification of participant volunteers (all professional backgrounds) from the team
3. Multi-professional training and skills development via a 2-day introductory workshop on solution-focused therapy for the participants
4. Open forums for SFI clinical supervision at 2-weekly intervals
5. Checklist for use in clinical practice formulated as a result of the supervision sessions
6. 2-day follow up workshop
7. Ongoing clinical supervision
8. Evaluation.

The evaluation emphasized the importance of solution-focused supervision, for both clinicians and managers. The need to assess the impact of introducing SFIs on team morale and individual stress levels was also identified; given the complexity of the client population this was key.

Following the evaluation, a multi-professional support group was developed, facilitated by an external person, to assist team members in managing their stress levels. Training in psychological therapy assessment skills across the team was initiated.

It should be noted SFT is now being used in the team's day-to-day practice, and is found to be relevant and effective, enhancing the confidence of clinicians to practise with a diverse client group. It has been adopted and promoted by the multidisciplinary team, including nurses and doctors, and has resulted in some positive patient outcomes. Moreover, it is worth noting that the experiences in this small local project have been further disseminated as a result of staff movement due to promotion, relocation or other development opportunity. At least three senior members of the team involved in doing this work have moved jobs and all three are actively involved in promoting this way of working, as appropriate, in new locations. Their positive experience in this project has clearly influenced their capacity to do this.

LESSONS ON GETTING RESEARCH INTO PRACTICE

It was interesting to note the parallels with this project and the action research approach described in Chapters 4 and 5. Although this was not formally set up as an action research approach, the features of assessing, planning and evaluating can be seen in the stages of the project. The ongoing support from a project facilitator played a part as did other aspects of this experience.

The recent literature indicates that mental health nurses are gradually becoming engaged in increasing numbers in the research process and are reporting the findings at national and international level. For research to become integral to practice the conditions noted in Table 9.2 are necessary. It can be seen that many of these could be applied to the local project introducing SFT discussed above.

In order to overcome the many barriers which prevent the integration of research into practice, Clifford & Murray (2001) stress the importance of collaborative approaches in which the project leader works in the clinical areas to ensure that staff have ownership of the research and that their strengths are valued and utilized.

Dodd (2001) suggests that mental health care has struggled with the notion of translating research into practice. Nevertheless, as the examples above show this can happen, but the impetus must be continued if mental health nursing is to grow in self-esteem and be able to provide person-centred care within an environment that values the people who come into contact with services.

The importance of integrating research into education and practice cannot be over-emphasized. It is clear from our experiences that clinical staff need support if they are to develop an environment in which research flourishes, both from the perspective of using existing knowledge (as in the SFI project), in collecting data to help us understand the care environment and

Table 9.2   Integrating research into practice

1. Research must be valued:
   - Beginning in the education process
   - Continuing through professional development
   - Research conducted that is real and relevant
   - Mental health nurses as active participants rather than subjects
2. Research must be integral:
   - To job descriptions
   - To individual performance review
   - To professional development
   - To clinical supervision
3. Resources and time must be available
   - Time must be allocated to research activity
   - IT resources must be available
   - Literature is required within the workplace
   - Time is needed for discussion

in taking a lead on other types of clinically-led research (see Ch. 6). It is suggested that the importance of having those with research training and skills visible within the clinical arena should not be underestimated and at this time those with expertise must be generous in supporting students and clinical staff who are keen to improve and evaluate their work. It is hoped that when researchers work regularly with clinical colleagues on research and development initiatives, the voice of the mental health nurse will be heard ever louder within the multidisciplinary team.

SUMMARY AND CONCLUSION

This brief overview of research in mental health nursing demonstrates that considerable progress has been made over the past few decades in terms of research activities. But research into practice is much more than merely doing research projects in practice, it is about the right research being done, it being owned by all concerned and the findings being valued and implemented. One finding that repeatedly surfaces in studies that aim to get research into practice is the importance of involving care providers at an early stage of the research. Their involvement is the key to ensuring that research is relevant and able to be implemented in practice.

REFERENCES

Altschul A 1972 Patient–nurse interactions: a study of interactive patterns in acute admission wards. Churchill Livingstone, Edinburgh
Barker P 1999 The philosophy and practice of psychiatric nursing. Churchill Livingstone, London
Barker P 2001 The tidal model: developing an empowering, person-centred approach to recovery within psychiatric and mental health nursing. Journal of Psychiatric and Mental Health Nursing 8: 233–240
Barker P 2002 Doing what needs to be done: a respectful response to Burnard and Grant. Journal of Psychiatric and Mental Health Nursing 9(2): 323
Barker P, Campbell P, Davidson B 1999 What are psychiatric nurses needed for? Developing a theory of essential nursing practice. Journal of Psychiatric and Mental Health Nursing 6: 273–282
Bowles N, Mackintosh C, Torn A 2001 Nurses' communication skills: an evaluation of the impact of solution-focused communication training. Journal of Advanced Nursing 36(3): 347–354
Burnard P 2002 Not waving but drowning: a personal response to Barker and Grant. Journal of Psychiatric and Mental Health Nursing 9: 230–233
Burnard P, Hannigan B 2000 Qualitative and quantitative approaches in mental health nursing: moving the debate forward. Journal of Psychiatric and Mental Health Nursing 7: 1–6
Cheek J 2000 Postmodern and poststructural approaches to nursing research. Sage, London
Clifford C, Murray S 2001 Pre- and post-test evaluation of a project to facilitate research development in practice in a hospital setting. Journal of Advanced Nursing 36(5): 685–695
Clinton M 1981 Training psychiatric nurses: a sociological study of the problem of integrating theory and practice. Unpublished PhD thesis, University of East Anglia
Cormack D 1976 Psychiatric nursing observed. Royal College of Nursing, London

Crawford P, Carr J, Knight A, Chambers K, Nolan P 2001 The value of community mental health nurses based in primary care teams: 'switching the light on in the cellar'. Journal of Psychiatric and Mental Health Nursing 8: 213–220

Davis B D 1986 A review of recent research in psychiatric nursing. In: Brooking J (ed) Psychiatric nursing research. John Wiley, Chichester

Department of Health 1991 The care programme approach. HMSO, London

Department of Health 1993 Working in partnership: a collaborative approach to care. Report of the Mental Health Nursing Review Team. HMSO, London

Department of Health 1999a National service framework for mental health. Stationery Office, London

Department of Health 1999b Making a difference. Stationery Office, London

Department of Health 2000 The NHS plan, a plan for investment, a plan for reform. Stationery Office, London

Department of Health 2001 Essence of care, benchmarking. Stationery Office, London

Department of Health and Social Security 1979 Organisational and management problems of mental illness hospitals: report of a working group [Nodder Report]. HMSO, London

Dodd H, Wellman N 2000 Staff development, anxiety and relaxation techniques: a pilot study in an acute psychiatric setting. Journal of Psychiatric and Mental Health Nursing 7(5): 443–448

Dodd T 2001 Clues about evidence for mental health care in community settings: assertive outreach. Mental Health Practice 4(7): 10–14

Dodds P, Bowles N 2001 Dismantling formal observation and refocusing nursing activity in acute inpatient psychiatry: a case study. Journal of Psychiatric and Mental Health Nursing 8(2): 183–188

Gallagher E B, Levinson D J, Ehrlich I 1957 Some socio-psychological characteristics of patients and their relevance for psychiatric treatment. In: Gallagher E B (ed) The patient and the mental hospital. Free Press, Glencoe

Gallop R 1998 Abuse of power in the nurse–client relationship. Nursing Standard 12(37): 43–47

Gournay K, Beardsmoore A 1995 The report of the Clinical Standards Advisory Group: standards of care for people with schizophrenia in the UK and implications for mental health nursing. Journal of Psychiatric and Mental Health Nursing 2: 359–364

Graham I W 2001 Seeking clarification of meaning: a phenomenological interpretation of the craft of mental health nursing. Journal of Psychiatric and Mental Health Nursing 8: 335–345

John A 1961 A study of the psychiatric nurse. E & S Livingstone, Edinburgh

Jorm A F 2000 Mental health literacy. British Journal of Psychiatry 177: 394–401

Liverpool Regional Hospital Board 1954 The work of mental nurses. Royal College of Psychiatrists, London

Maddox M 1957 The work of mental nurses. Nursing Mirror 105: 189–190

Manchester Regional Hospital Board 1956 The work of the mental nurse. Royal College of Psychiatrists, London

Martin J P 1984 Hospitals in trouble. Basic Blackwell, London

Mental Health Act Commission 1997 The national visit. HMSO, London

Merwin E, Mauck A 1995 Psychiatric nursing research: the state of the science. Journal of Psychiatric Nursing 9(6): 311–331

Nolan P 1995 The development of mental health nursing. In: Carson J, Fagin L, Ritter S (eds) Stress and coping in mental health nursing. Chapman and Hall, London

Nolan P, Haque M, Badger F, Dyke R, Khan I 2001 Mental health nurses' perceptions of nurse prescribing. Journal of Advanced Nursing 36(4): 527–534

O'Connell B 1998 Solution-focused therapy. Sage, London

Oppenheim A M, Ereman B 1955 The function and training of mental nurses. Chapman and Hall, London

Owen S 2001 The practical, methodological and ethical dilemmas of conducting focus groups with vulnerable clients. Journal of Advanced Nursing 36(5): 652–658

Pollock L C 1982 Community psychiatric nursing: myth and reality. Royal College of Nursing, London

Psychiatric Nursing Today and Tomorrow 1968 Report of the joint sub-committee of the standing mental health and standing nursing advisory committees. HMSO, London

Sainsbury Centre for Mental Health 2001 Acute concerns and acute solutions. Briefing Papers 4, 5. Sainsbury Centre, London

Schon D 1983 The reflective practitioner. Basic Books, New York

Taylor R, Coombes L, Bartlett H 2002 The impact of a practice development project on the quality of inpatient small group therapy. Journal of Psychiatric and Mental Health Nursing 9: 213–220

Towell D 1975 Understanding psychiatric nursing. Royal College of Nursing, London

Wales P 1998 Solution-focused brief therapy in primary care. Nursing Times 94(15): 48–49

Wilgosh R, Hawkes D, Marsh I 1992 Focusing on solutions. Nursing Times 88(31): 46–48

10

Undertaking feasibility studies in primary care

Paramjit S. Gill   David Jones

Editors' comment

In this chapter the focus is on 'doing research'. The authors, both general practitioners, have given a clear account of some of the practical issues involved in designing and developing a research project in primary care. In this chapter the authors have illustrated clearly the challenges faced when wanting to develop a service that is based upon research findings. The account of a quasi-experimental study, that was seen as a pilot study for larger scale activity, illustrates the challenges researchers face if they want their work to stand up to rigorous scrutiny in the research community. The authors demonstrate that it is the research question that should drive the research and how, in undertaking a pragmatic research (that is real world research), adjustments have to be made to methodological ideology. Textbook descriptions of research processes can sometimes imply that experimental approaches to research are simple if certain steps are taken. However, this is not always such a straightforward process, and this chapter gives a good example of some of the challenges in setting up even a relatively small feasibility study.

INTRODUCTION

In this chapter we provide an overview of conducting research within primary care. We highlight pertinent issues by drawing on the phases of the research cycle and our own study.

The history of research within general practice and primary care started nearly 200 years ago. A number of general practitioners (GPs) have made substantial contributions to medical knowledge. Notably, two of these practitioners provided vital insight into the epidemiology of infectious diseases: Jenner found that cowpox provided protection against smallpox (RCGP 1992) and Budd showed that typhoid was spread by water (Budd 1873).

In the 20th century valuable contributions were made by many GPs, including Mackenzie (1916), Pickles (1939), Fry (1966), Tudor Hart (1980) and Crombie (1963). All of these practitioner-researchers worked initially within their own practices. It was not until 1957 that the first university department of general practice was established in Edinburgh.

Why do research in primary care?

The term primary care is used here to reflect front line care in first contact with the public, and the major part of primary care in the UK is general practice based: that is a team of healthcare practitioners usually led by a medically qualified doctor, the GP. The major strength of general practice is that about 97% of the population is registered with a GP (RCGP 1990) and that patients stay registered with the same GP for an average of 12 years thereby providing continuity of care (Howie et al 1997). Further, GPs manage the majority of problems within primary care and act as 'gate-keeper' to specialist services such as those provided within the hospital – or secondary care – service. Consequently, GPs are in a unique position to deal with the early diagnosis and prevention of important, common problems that impinge upon individuals and their families (Howie et al 1997, Mant 1997).

In the past there were many barriers for individual practitioners to actively undertake research including:

- Isolation – many practitioners with a research interest worked alone
- Service commitment with a high workload
- Resources in terms of time and funding
- No career structure
- Motivation.

During the last decade there has been a major shift in policy with an emphasis on evidence-based culture particularly within primary care (see Chs 2, 3 and 5). Recommendations from a raft of reports highlight the need for increasing research capacity within primary care with adequate training, increasing funding and development of transparent arrangements, establishment of research networks and research practices (Carter et al 2001). This is in partnership with university departments of general practice and local providers and is now much more likely to include all members of the healthcare team.

The Royal College of General Practitioners (RCGP) has contributed to research within primary care by establishing the Birmingham Research Unit in 1959 (Fleming 2001) and the Manchester Research Unit in 1968 (Hannaford 2001). Both of these units continue to make major contributions to research within primary care. The college also facilitates and supports research in a number of ways: for example the establishment of the RCGP master classes in primary care; research fellowships; and research funding which is open to other disciplines but where priority is given to practising GPs and other members of the primary healthcare team (see http://www.rcgp.org.uk/rcgp/webmaster/research_sub.asp).

RESEARCH CYCLE

Previous chapters have highlighted the issues to consider in undertaking research and this can be viewed as a research cycle (Fig. 10.1). We will use the research cycle to highlight a number of issues that arose in this research, which involved two GPs.

The idea or subject area

The cycle starts with the idea that may be worth investigating. Ideas arise mainly from one's own practice, as GPs are in a unique position where they see over 60% of their practice population in a year. Many problems are raised during the consultation. In our case we both practise in highly diverse urban areas where there are large numbers of refugees, and identified a lack of adequate interpreting services to provide effective healthcare to our practice population.

As with any problem, especially one involving different intellectual domains, it is best to discuss the issues with colleagues, local academic departments of general practice and experts within the field (see Chs 1 and 12). We felt that the problem of overcoming language barriers in medicine was

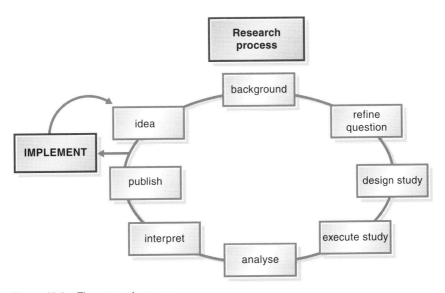

Figure 10.1   The research process.

such a major issue involving questions about migration, equity, economic resources and availability of technology within the health service that we wrote an editorial (Jones & Gill 1998). This process helped us to clarify the issues and move on to the next phase of the research process: the background.

BACKGROUND

By reviewing the literature and contacting colleagues and experts we were able to provide the evidence base in this area. This was done using a quasi-experimental research approach. Here an experimental method may be seen as the ideal design but it is not possible to achieve one or more of the three criteria for experimental design, namely randomization, control and manipulation.

Randomization means that 'every member of a given population' is given a chance to participate; manipulation means that the researcher controls the research interventions that are being studied (i.e. the independent variable); control means that any variables that might influence the measurement of the impact of the intervention (dependent variables) are managed or at least considered (Clifford 1997). In an ideal experimental design the researcher will achieve the optimal level of experimental design if s/he is 'blind' to the research intervention when measuring the impact of the intervention. Such a scenario can be achieved, for example, in healthcare research in drug trials when neither the prescribing doctor nor the patient knows whether they are receiving a trial drug (independent variable) when the doctor is measuring the impact of the drug (dependant variable). This is known as a 'double-blind' study. Here, as will be seen below, it was not possible to 'blind' the researchers or the participants to the activities in this study although clear attempts were made to manipulate the independent variable and consider aspects that impacted upon the dependant variables.

There is a growing need in the UK to provide readily accessible and appropriate interpreting services for the diverse population who use the NHS. The number of different languages spoken by non-English-speaking patients in metropolitan areas presents a formidable obstacle and this diversity of languages is a particular challenge as provision of physically present interpreters for all languages spoken is not possible. This may be due to a lack of interpreters in the area or, most importantly, simple lack of resources to have staff available just in case they are needed. It is worth noting that the total cost of providing an interpreter for a single brief consultation in this way usually includes a much larger element for travel time. Provision of physically present interpreters for all possible languages, 24 hours a day, in all health settings appears to be unrealistic.

As stated above, the majority of healthcare contacts take place in general practice and GPs in inner cities can often obtain a professional interpreter for consultations that may be classed as 'important', for example, because of preliminary knowledge of the patient's condition – but what of consultations that are not planned in advance? The provision of a full-time on-site interpreter is feasible and affordable when there is sufficient need to provide interpreting in a single language. Only practices with a majority of patients from a single language community can expect to have an interpreter available throughout surgery hours. The much more typical inner-city practice, with small numbers of non-English-speaking patients from several language communities, is likely to have very limited access to professional interpreting.

Healthcare professionals then must choose between several imperfect alternatives including using the patient's friends, relatives or children. In the USA published guidelines for language services in a health context strongly caution against the use of informal interpreters (Perkins et al 1998). There are concerns about confidentiality and about the accuracy of informal interpreters. Although children lack the emotional and cognitive maturity to assume the responsibility of interpreting conversations between parents and professionals they are often used in this role (Jones & Gill 1998). The lack of interpreting services for non-English-speaking patients presenting acutely is a source of real danger for the patient and adds significantly to the stress experienced by the clinician and the informal interpreter.

This is a really important issue for ill patients who may find it impossible to access primary care as even making an appointment at a GP surgery can be problematic. In such cases, patients may choose to attend the local accident and emergency department as they perceive this as the only alternative, for in such departments staff are required to undertake health assessments and determine a line of treatment as appropriate. While this may mean the patient's needs are met, it is not necessarily the most cost-efficient way of providing for care needs.

Remote interpreting

Remote interpreting is described as a situation where an interpreter is based at a central location and can be accessed via a telephone line. This is a system that can be used when a physically present interpreter is not available or when resources for a physically present interpreter cannot be justified because the number of non-English-speaking patients is too small (Pointon 1996, Jones & Gill 1998).

We believe that remote interpreting will prove to be a very cost-effective way for interpreters to provide a flexible service over a very large geographical area. The creation of a centrally located pool of interpreters who can be accessed remotely also opens up the possibility of a more rational use of available languages skills including the pooling of resources from different agencies. However, the NHS still needs to be persuaded that remote interpreting offers a solution to the challenge created by linguistic diversity as evidence generated by research to address this issue is lacking.

In the UK, commercial telephone translation services are available but are expensive, and employ interpreters who may not have experience in interpreting in a health setting. Further, where NHS trusts offer local telephone interpreting services provision is often patchy. Little is known in the UK about the effects of different translation provision on the quality or costs of healthcare, but evidence from the USA suggests that it can allow high-quality consultations and is valued by patients (Hornberger 1998). Remote access to interpreters using a telephone line has been used but has been criticized on the grounds that non-verbal aspects of communication are unavailable to the interpreter (Levinson & Gillam 1998), yet it may be the only practical way of providing professional interpreting in acute clinical situations (Leman 1997).

During the last 10 years technology has been developed to use video-conferencing within the healthcare setting (Harrison et al 1996). The use of tele-medicine technology to provide remote interpreting in language discordant consultations between patient and doctor is a significant innovation. The practical problems of this new application of video-conferencing technology remain unexplored.

RESEARCH QUESTION

The background reading in this area helped us to clarify the research question. A good research question has to be important to *you*, interesting, and capable of being answered within a relatively short time period (Howie 1989). It should also bear in mind resource issues. We were certain that the first step would be to do a feasibility study before embarking on a large study. This would ensure that this intervention was feasible within routine general practice; raise any logistic issues; and provide help with sample size estimation for the larger study. This is common practice in developing health services research as there would be little value in supporting research activity on a larger scale if in reality it would not be possible to undertake the work proposed. In many research texts the notion of a feasibility study is often omitted or referred to very fleetingly in the context of discussions about a 'pilot' study. The way in which a feasibility study differs from a pilot study is that it does not assume at the outset the work will be progressed; that will only happen if the initial idea does lend itself to further research. In the study proposed here it was not known at the outset whether the ideas generated by the researchers could be carried through to practice so it was important to test this out before proposing any larger-scale work. Clearly, if the idea could not be researched well following the methodology planned it would be necessary to review our proposals and look at other ways of examining this issue (see alternative approaches in Ch. 5).

So our question was: is it feasible to develop remote interpreting, including the application of tele-medicine technology for non-English-speaking patients, within routine general practice?

METHODS

A quasi-randomized study design was chosen, as a double-blind randomized control study was not feasible at this stage. The remote interpreting services (i.e. the independent variables) and the outcome measures (the dependant variables) are described below.

Study population

We chose Turkish-speaking patients consulting the GP who needed interpreting services as this specific group is a reflection of the population of non-English speakers registered at one of the author's (DJ) practice. Selection of a single language community limits the resources (in terms of interpreter time) required for a small-scale feasibility study. We hoped that the information gained from this feasibility study would be sufficiently applicable to the general problem of language discordant consultations to contribute significantly to the methodology of a future intervention study involving several different language communities.

To examine this within our chosen methodology we wanted to compare the impact of interpreting services using several approaches. We aimed to recruit 10–12 patients using each of the following interpreting methods:

* Interpreter physically present with GP
* Interpreter available via remote telephone without visual link
* Interpreter available in remote location using a visual link via telemedicine technology.

Setting

This project was located in one GP surgery and DJ ran these sessions in his practice. To manage this, 3-hour surgery sessions with dedicated GP time at 30-minute intervals were booked. The interpreters were available during this time either with the GP, via a telephone link, or via a video link.

The remote interpreter was accessed using a dedicated ISDN or telephone line. The ISDN simulator link was to an on-site interpreter located in another room in the health centre. The length of the consultation was recorded and the GP also recorded the principal diagnosis as well as basic demographic information.

Outcome measures

To determine if new approaches to care do make a difference within experimental design, it is important to be very clear about exactly what is being measured. This is referred to as the outcome measure. The outcome measures are used to analyse the impact of the research intervention. The aim is to be able to state with confidence that the measures are giving an accurate representation of the impact of the research intervention. So, for example, if a dietician was recommending a new diet to help weight loss in an obese patient a simple outcome measure would be weight loss.

In a study such as this which was focusing on the acceptability of a new technique, including the application of tele-medicine technology for non-English-speaking patients within routine general practice, finding the right outcome measures was another challenge to the researchers. To do this the following outcome measures were used in the study:

1. The Patient Enablement Instrument (PEI) (Howie et al 1999). This is designed to measure the degree to which the patient has been enabled by the consultation to understand and cope with their condition. The scores range from 0 to 12 with high scores indicating high levels of enablement.

2. A 21-question version of the Medical Interview Satisfaction Scale (MISS21) questionnaire (Wolf et al 1978, Wolf & Stiles 1981). This is designed to measure patient satisfaction with individual consultations in UK general practice. It provides a measure of satisfaction with ease of communication (Communication Comfort subscale), the emotional content of the consultation (Rapport subscale), relief of concerns (Distress Relief subscale) and prescribed treatment (Compliance Intent subscale) as well as an overall measure of satisfaction. The score ranges between 1 and 7, with 7 indicating the highest level of satisfaction.

3. All patients completed four further questions designed to explore patients' perceptions of the quality of communication and degree of discomfort with the interpreting process and sense of well-being following the consultation. Patients allocated a telephone interpreter were asked a further question about sound quality. Patients allocated a video interpreter were asked about sound and picture quality. Patients allocated to both telephone and video conferencing were also asked if they would be prepared to use these techniques again. None of the 11 patients allocated a video conferencing interpreter had previous experience of this technique and they were invited to compare video conferencing with 'other types of interpreting service' by responding to a further question.

Translating the tools used

Before using the above instruments we had to validate them for use among Turkish-speakers as these instruments were originally developed and validated for English-speakers only. The instruments were translated into Turkish and back-translated independently into English by a second interpreter using current guidelines (Fitzpatrick et al 1998, Gill & Jones 2000). A commercial agency was used for this process.

The Turkish translation obtained was explored further by a focus group of Turkish-speaking bilingual healthcare workers and monolingual non-English-speaking Turkish participants for face and content validity. The groups were recruited from the participating health centre. The focus group was tape-recorded and the translation was modified and returned to the independent translator. The resulting translation was again explored by the focus group and a final version agreed (Brislin 1970).

Semi-structured interviews

To obtain a range of views on interpreting services we randomly selected four subjects from each group for interview. Participants were encouraged to discuss their last interpreting method and to reflect on their past experiences of interpreting. The interviews were conducted by PG with help from another interpreter, in the participants' homes, and lasted up to 30 minutes. The interviews were audio-taped, and all the English language sections transcribed before analysis.

Ethical approval and consent

At the start of any study it is important to obtain ethical approval from the local research ethics committee and get written consent from all participants. Note that new arrangements are now in place so that you do not have to submit to more than one committee for approval (see http://www.corec.org.uk/). This stage can also take time so do plan well in advance and pay particular attention to letters informing potential subjects about your study. We obtained both verbal and written consent using a consent form that, like the research instruments, had been translated and back-translated into Turkish. This was very important for it was essential that those patients participating in the feasibility study knew what they were agreeing to do. For those involved in the video component the visual link was not switched on until written informed consent was obtained.

Doing the study

Funding and timescale are vital aspects. Funding of research is an important issue and many opportunities exist within primary care to undertake small-scale feasibility studies with primary care. However, for those new to research it is important not to underestimate the cost required to set up a relatively small feasibility study such as this. Obvious costs include the GP's and interpreter's time both for the consultations and for the data collection described. In the description above other aspects can be readily identified. For example the cost of the video link and the telephone link. The costs of translations feature highly in this project as does the need to cost the instruments used for data collection (if there is a charge for these) and the analysis. Not stated here but also worthy of consideration is the need to consider the cost of the 'next steps'. For example, it is noted below (Dissemination) that we have written a report of our activities for publication and have prepared a bid for further funding for a larger-scale project. All these things take time and effort so must be considered at the outset.

There are a number of sources of funding for research in primary care. Some of the funders include primary care networks (Hungin 1999) and the RCGP Scientific Foundation (http://www.rcgp.org.uk/rcgp/research/ sci_foundationboard/sfb_index.asp). We obtained funding for this study from the North Thames Primary Care Network (http://www.ucl.ac.uk/ primcare-popsci/nocten/) (see also Ch. 2 re NHS research funding).

Another important aspect not to underestimate is how much time it takes to get even a relatively small feasibility study completed. The whole process reported here took about 12 months to complete. This highlights the importance of being realistic with project milestones. Planning a project timetable is essential and will pay dividends later as it highlights key development points and areas to consider for the successful completion of a study.

One area where we underestimated the time involved was to do with translation of our questionnaire into Turkish. We approached a commercial organization that promised to translate and back-translate independently following established guidelines (Gill & Jones 2000). Unfortunately this process took over 6 months mainly due to professional translators not agreeing on the text! Once we had the translated version we then went to a focus group of Turkish-speakers and this further extended our timetable. This was an important aspect as the validity of the study depended on this.

We also failed to realize how difficult it would be to fix sessions with the interpreters as they only worked during specified hours. Further, the hardware had to be installed within the practice and this took 6 weeks in total.

Once the equipment had been installed, the GP (DJ) had to have some training on using it within the consultation. This was arranged with the local department of general practice.

It is worth noting here that the team involvement in this study was contained within general practice, interpreting and technical services involved in setting up systems and translating the instruments used. When considering project development do consider how much more complex it might have been had this stage of study involved other members of the primary care team, perhaps by introducing interpretative services into the practice nurse or allied health professional clinics in the healthcare centre involved.

The above points highlight the importance of time as a resource as the research study had to fit within existing service commitments. One can never plan for too much time to think, execute, interpret and write up the study.

Analysis and interpretation of data

The researchers involved in this study were experienced in data analysis and so this aided this aspect of the research. New researchers will undoubtedly need help in this aspect and this reinforces the point made above about working with local academic providers to help with analysis.

Quantitative data were entered into a database and analysed using SPSS software. For the qualitative data, to maximize reliability and validity, all reports were read and themed independently by both of us using the technique of charting which involved reading and re-reading the transcripts and independently selecting and reorganizing responses according to themes. Both of us then met and agreed on the themes and any disagreement was resolved by discussion (Bryman & Burgess 1994).

Dissemination

Once all data were analysed and interpreted, the final stage involved disseminating the findings. This is important so that key messages are widely publicized through as many outlets as possible, such as at local meetings; conferences (Jones et al 2003a); and in peer reviewed journals (Jones et al 2003b). This not only adds to the evidence base in this area but also, hopefully, leads to implementation of the findings.

We found that both video conferencing and hands-free telephones can deliver an acceptable interpreting service within primary care. From our interviews the following themes emerged:

1. Ready availability of interpreting is crucial
2. Use of relatives as interpreters is often, but not always, unacceptable
3. Patients are reluctant to express a preference for a particular interpreting method
4. Some patients preferred the video conferencing to the telephone
5. Video conferencing can create a 'camera shy' response.

Writing for peer reviewed journals is a time-consuming activity and you will need to set aside some time for this. This is usually underestimated and when seeking funding it is vital to cost this into the proposal. The results of this particular study have been submitted to a peer reviewed journal and funding is being sought to continue with the larger trial.

SUMMARY AND CONCLUSION

This chapter has offered an outline of an experience of undertaking a research project in primary care. The study was designed to improve the quality of care given to a specific minority group – i.e. Turkish people – accessing GP services in one locality. It has been used to illustrate some of the practical issues that can arise in setting up and developing a research study. A small feasibility study was chosen for this purpose as it demonstrates that a couple of practitioners working together with the aid or appropriate support from primary care research networks and an academic department in a university can undertake worthwhile research that can lead to a larger scale project being developed.

The time and resource issues involved in this research are important to note as this indicates what may be feasible to do within the bounds of every-day practice and the level of research that might require the involvement of a much larger team. We have, for example, noted that in this feasibility project we chose to work with only one minority group as this would be easier given the procedures we wanted to develop and test. We also indicated that if the feasibility study proved successful, then we would wish to expand the research to a greater number of minority groups and to a larger number of GP practices. For those new to research a simple calculation multiplying the time taken for the one minority group studied here by a higher number of minority groups in your own geographical location and the number of GP surgeries that could be involved in different locations in different parts of the country gives an indication of the scale of a full study in both time and resources.

We have found that patience and planning are the vital elements for con-ducting research within primary care. We have learned to value the model of developing a feasibility study before making a full commitment to pro-jects such as this that may be complex in both design and delivery and as such strongly recommend that all research in primary care is subject to the same careful processes.

ACKNOWLEDGEMENTS

The study was funded by the North Central Thames Primary Care Research Network (NoCTeN). We thank all participants for taking part in this study and Semra Ahmet, Konce Sah and Arzu Kaya for providing the interpreting service.

REFERENCES

Brislin R 1970 Back-translation for cross-cultural research. Journal of Cross-cultural Psychology 3: 185–216
Bryman A, Burgess R G (eds) 1994 Analysing qualitative data. Routledge, London
Budd W 1873 Typhoid fever. Longmans Green, London
Carter Y, Elwyn G, Hungin P (eds) 2001 General practitioner research at the millennium: a perspective from the RCGP. Royal College of General Practitioners, London
Clifford C 1997 Nursing and health care research. Prentice-Hall, London
Crombie D L 1963 The defects of general practice. Lancet 1: 209–211
Fitzpatrick R, Davey C, Buxton M J, Jones D R 1998 Evaluating patient-based outcome measures for use in clinical trials. Health Technology Assessment 2(14): i–iv, 1–74

Fleming D 2001 A review of the Birmingham Research Unit. In: Carter Y, Elwyn G, Hungin P (eds) General practitioner research at the millennium: a perspective from the RCGP. Royal College of General Practitioners, London

Fry J 1966 A study in the natural history of common diseases. E&S Livingstone, Edinburgh

Gill P S, Jones D 2000 Cross-cultural adaptation of outcome measures. European Journal of General Practice 6: 120–121

Hannaford P 2001 The RCGP Centre for Primary Care Research and Epidemiology. In: Carter Y, Elwyn G, Hungin P (eds) General practitioner research at the millennium: a perspective from the RCGP. Royal College of General Practitioners, London

Harrison R, Clayton W, Wallace P 1996 Can telemedicine be used to improve communication between primary and secondary care? British Medical Journal 313: 1377–1380

Hornberger J 1998 Evaluating the cost of bridging language barriers in health care. Journal of Health Care for the Poor and Underserved 9: S26–S39

Howie J G R 1989 Research in general practice. Chapman and Hall, London

Howie J G R, Heaney D J, Maxwell M 1997 Measuring quality in general practice. Occasional Paper no. 75. Royal College of General Practitioners, London

Howie J, Heaney D, Maxwell M, Walker J, Freeman G, Rai H 1999. Quality at general practice consultations: cross sectional survey. British Medical Journal 319: 738–743

Hungin P 1999 Research networks. In: Carter Y, Thomas C (eds) Research opportunities in primary care. Radcliffe Medical Press, Oxford

Jones D, Gill P 1998 Breaking down language barriers. British Medical Journal 316: 1476

Jones D, Gill P, Harrison R, Wallace P 2003a Videoconferencing for remote interpretation in the general practice consultation: an exploratory study. Telemedicine 2003: 10th Anniversary International Conference on Telemedicine and Telecare. Royal Society of Medicine, London, 29–30 January

Jones D, Gill P, Harrison R, Meakin R, Wallace P 2003b Videoconferencing for remote interpretation in the general practice consultation – an exploratory study. Journal of Telemedicine and Telecare 9: 51–56

Leman P 1997 Interpreter use in an inner city accident and emergency department. Journal of Accident and Emergency Medicine 14: 98–100

Levinson R, Gillam S 1998 Linkworkers in primary care. King's Fund Primary Care Series. King's Fund Publishing, London

Mackenzie J 1916 Principles of diagnosis and treatment in heart affections. Henry Frowde and Hodder and Stoughton, London

Mant D 1997 R&R in primary care: National Working Group report. Department of Health, Leeds

Perkins J, Simon H, Cheng F, Olsen K, Vera Y 1998 Ensuring linguistic access in health care settings: legal rights and responsibilities: Henry J Kaiser Family Foundation, California

Pickles W 1939 Epidemiology in country practice. John Wright, Bristol

Pointon T 1996 Telephone interpreting service is available. British Medical Journal 312: 53

Royal College of General Practitioners 1992 Forty years on: the story of the first forty years of the Royal College of General Practitioners. Royal College of General Practitioners, London

Royal College of General Practitioners 1990 A college plan: priorities for the future. Occasional Paper no. 49. Royal College of General Practitioners, London

Tudor Hart J 1980 Hypertension. Churchill Livingstone, Edinburgh

Wolf M H, Stiles W B 1981 Further development of the medical interview satisfaction scale. A paper presented at the American Psychological Association Convention, Los Angeles, CA

Wolf M H, Putnam S M, James A J, Stiles W B 1978 The medical interview satisfaction scale: development of a scale to measure patient perceptions of physician behaviour. Journal of Behavioral Medicine 1: 391–401

A personal journey

Carol Dealey

INTRODUCTION

Up until the mid 1980s, nursing expertise in wound management tended to centre around skills in undertaking dressing change, using what was often described as 'a good aseptic technique'. The advent of new theories in wound management and a wide variety of wound management products resulted in wound management becoming more complex. At the same time there was increasing awareness of the problem of pressure ulcers and the importance of good prevention strategies. Nurses became aware of the need for advice and support in wound management which ultimately resulted in the first clinical nurse specialist (CNS) in tissue viability being appointed in 1987 (Dealey 1988). Tissue viability can be defined as the management and prevention of wounds of all aetiologies. In the UK, the development of tissue viability as a specialty has been very much led by nurses with limited interest from other healthcare professionals.

In the early years there was considerable pressure from senior managers in many hospitals to justify the need for a CNS post. There was also a lack of both theoretical and clinical knowledge to support CNSs in their role. Thus, there was a need for research to supply guidance for best practice in this area of work.

This chapter explores the development of a research base to underpin clinical practice from the perspective of one of the first nurses to become a clinical nurse specialist in tissue viability. Some of the drivers for research will be discussed as well as the challenges in undertaking research in the clinical arena. Although the author has undertaken research in relation to several wound types, for the purposes of clarity only research relating to the prevention and management of pressure ulcers will be used as exemplars in this chapter. Each exemplar will describe the background to the research study, the methods and results and the learning about research that occurred.

The research discussed in this chapter is based on some of the work undertaken by the author during a 12-year period, mostly while working as a CNS in tissue viability in an elderly care hospital and also in an acute teaching hospital. The experience gained from this research paved the way for the author's current role as a research lead in a teaching hospital setting. The learning by experience described below is now being used to help others develop their knowledge and insights into research while, hopefully, avoiding a number of the pitfalls described below.

AN INDIVIDUAL JOURNEY INTO RESEARCH DEVELOPMENT

Research is undertaken for a variety of reasons. From the perspective of this author, several drivers impacted upon the research journey in which she learned about research. They are described as:

- Internal: personal and professional views that lead to research questions
- External: pressure to measure or justify situations

Table 11.1 Drivers on the research journey

Personal driver – *What is best practice in the prevention and management of pressure ulcers?*
Research questions
  How bad is the problem of pressure ulcers in my hospital?
  What are the specific problems for my group of patients?
  What is the most appropriate mattress/overlay for different patient groups?
  What are the most appropriate dressings for use on pressure ulcers?

External drivers – *Pressures to justify CNS role or the need to purchase equipment*
Research studies
  Calculating the cost of treating pressure ulcers
  Evaluations of armchairs for patients at risk of pressure ulcer development

Personal experience – *The impact of undertaking research*
Outcomes
  Greater rigour in undertaking research
  Better use of statistics

Opportunistic drivers – *External requests to undertake research generally commercially funded*
Research studies
  Evaluation of pressure relieving equipment
  Comparative study of two wound management products

- Personal experience: developing skills in research which lead to more appropriate selection of methodologies and greater rigour in the research process
- Opportunistic: requests to undertake research studies – generally commercially funded.

Examples of these drivers can be found in Table 11.1.

It must be acknowledged that it is only with the advantage of hindsight that these drivers can be recognized. At the time it seemed that as one question was answered, more research questions were identified, leading to further research. There was no pre-planned strategy; the sustaining driving force was a desire to give patients the best care possible. If there was insufficient research to identify 'best practice', then it was an indication to undertake further research. Unfortunately, this lack of a pre-planned strategy can result in changes in patterns of data collection over time, which result in poor data and, in turn, impact on the quality of longitudinal evidence available (Dealey 2000).

Serendipity can also have a role in research. One example is when the author was approached to undertake an evaluation of a seat specifically designed for patients with seating difficulties. The request came about a week after a survey of the chairs in the hospital had been completed. This local work had shown that a number of patients were placed in chairs in a very poor state of repair simply because they were unable to sit in ordinary chairs. The opportunity to evaluate new seating was timely for this group of people although of course the evaluative study had to be very carefully designed to avoid the bias that could have occurred through simply improving the seating.

The next section will present a series of exemplars that give brief accounts of a number of studies the author was involved in in the early days of her research experience.

Exemplar 11.1

Background

The principle reason for establishing the role of CNS in tissue viability was to establish appropriate strategies for the prevention and management of pressure ulcers. It was therefore logical that measuring the size of the problem should be identified as a first step. This required a review of the extent to which pressure sores were a problem in the hospital in which the CNS worked.

Methods and results

The research method used was that of a point prevalence survey. Point prevalence can be defined as: 'The number of persons with a specific disease or condition as a proportion of a given population, measured at a specific point in time' (Dealey 1997). Thus, for example, a point prevalence survey of pressure ulcers in one hospital could be defined as: 'The number of patients in Royal Hospital with pressure ulcers, as a proportion of the total number of in-patients, measured on 1st September.'

A prevalence survey can be used to collect more data than just the numbers of pressure ulcers. It is important, for example, to collect information about the grade and positions of the ulcers. It can also be useful to collect information about the level of risk of each patient within the population to be measured, the type of mattress they have on their beds and which dressings are being used on the pressure ulcers. Such information can be used to answer a number of questions:

- How many patients have pressure ulcers?
- What grade are they?
- What position are they on the body?
- What is the level of risk of pressure ulcer development for patients in the hospital?
- What type of mattresses are available and are they being used appropriately?
- Are suitable dressings being selected to treat pressure ulcers and are they in the hospital formulary?

Two papers were subsequently published (Dealey 1991, 1994a) to show how this type of information was collected within a series of pressure ulcer surveys.

Key aspects included ensuring the work was shared with all key stakeholders. At the planning stage, the author ensured support for the surveys by attending meetings held by ward sisters/charge nurses to explain the value of collecting the data. This was a crucial stage both in informing clinical staff about the purpose of the research and in gaining cooperation in the next phase, the data collection.

To facilitate the data collection it was agreed that a 'link' nurse from each ward or unit was appointed to organize the data collection in their area. An important aspect of research is to ensure that data collected in an observational study is consistent. Given this it was important to be quite explicit about the type of data that would be collected and to develop strategies for doing this in a consistent manner even though it was a team of nurses, rather than an individual, collecting the data. To address this the link nurses attended one of a series of training meetings held to provide standardized information about all aspects of the study.

A third key dimension was to ensure consistency in the sample group, the in-patients who were to be included in the survey. Clearly only patients with pressure sores were to be included and it was agreed that if they were in-patients at 0600 hours on the day of the survey they would be included. Thus the survey included all those being discharged from the hospital that day but excluded all admissions.

Discussion
Comparison with other prevalence surveys must be undertaken only with caution. The populations in one acute hospital may be quite different from another, for example there may or may not be maternity beds catering for a population of younger, commonly healthy women who are less likely to be at risk of pressure sores. It makes more sense to compare prevalence surveys in one hospital over time, although the results must be treated with caution if the patient population alters considerably (Dealey 2000). It may also be helpful to compare the findings of a survey with national surveys. The Dutch undertake annual prevalence surveys, which allow year-on-year comparisons of both the overall figures and also the prevalence in different categories of care providers (Bours et al 1999).

Research lessons learned from this study
A lot was learned in undertaking this work in terms of communicating information about projects and developing a shared commitment to data collection which was, after all, being undertaken to help develop better care for patients. As a result of the series of surveys undertaken, the information obtained was used to develop strategies for the selection of appropriate equipment to meet patient needs. Patterns that were identified in terms of care provision also indicated areas of knowledge deficit and poor practice among the nursing staff and so enabled the CNS to work with other key staff to plan appropriate education programmes.

Exemplar 11.2

Background
The methodology used in the prevalence surveys described in Exemplar 11.1 included a risk assessment of every patient in the hospital, using the Waterlow

score (Waterlow 1985). The hospital population could then be grouped into no risk, low risk, high risk and very high risk categories. For example, in one study, 12% of patients were at very high risk of developing pressure ulcers (Dealey 1991).

Identification of the level of risk of patients in the hospitals raised awareness of the need for an adequate amount of appropriate pressure redistributing equipment. This concern was exacerbated by an audit of the existing mattresses in both hospitals that had revealed that many were in urgent need of replacement. The management team in the elderly care hospital was prepared to undertake a gradual replacement of the mattresses. Most of the mattress stock comprised NHS mattresses, many of which were thought to be considerably older than the recommended lifespan of 4 years. They were also not considered suitable for patients at risk of pressure ulcer development because the foam was too shallow.

In 1989, the Vaperm™ mattress was considered to be a suitable alternative to older style provision in hospital (Scales et al 1982) and had been reported to have a lifespan of up to 9 years (Lowthian 1989). It should be noted that the evidence base for these conclusions was very limited, but a decision still had to be made as to how to replace worn out mattresses and there was little evidence upon which to make this decision. A mattress replacement programme purchasing Vaperm™ mattresses was successfully instigated at the elderly care hospital. However, no such monies were forthcoming in the acute hospital because this was not seen to be a priority at that time. It is interesting to note the difference in priorities between the two hospitals, which, it could be suggested, resulted in inequity of care provision at that time. It should be noted that some years later funding for mattress replacement was finally established in the acute hospital. This experience showed how managerial decisions could impact upon the ideology of implementing research. However, it should also be noted that this work was undertaken before the evidence-based practice movement was introduced (see Chs 2 and 3) and it may be surmised that a different outcome would be noted in today's culture.

Back in 1990, however, this lack of funding for mattress replacement in the acute hospital resulted in the need to develop alternative strategies. Thus, requests to undertake commercially funded research were seen as opportunities to obtain equipment. Serendipity appeared to step in again as an opportunity arose in 1990 to evaluate Vaperm™ mattresses within the acute hospital. This came about because changes in the law regarding fire retardancy meant that a combustion modified foam had to be used instead of the original foam in all mattresses (Dealey 1992). Some of the early versions of the combustion modified foam had collapsed within a few months of being used. Ultimately, the manufacturers developed a version of the foam that was considered to be more durable and comfortable than the original combustion modified foam. The proposed study was to compare the two types of foam.

Methods and results

The study was a double blind study (see Ch. 10) in that the researcher was aware that she had been supplied with 10 mattresses of each type of foam, but did not know which was which. The ward nurses were not aware of any difference between the mattresses. The underside of 10 mattresses were marked with an X indicating that they all had the same foam, but this was done by the manufacturer. The other 10 mattresses were left unmarked. Two of each type of mattress were distributed to five wards for a 12-month evaluation of normal usage. The ward nurses were advised that the mattresses were suitable for patients at moderate risk of pressure ulcer development. The patients using the mattresses were to be audited each week by the ward staff in respect of pressure ulcer risk and the presence/absence of pressure ulcers. The researcher tested the mattresses each month for 'grounding' (that is, collapse of the foam so that the bed base can be felt through it). Patient and nurse questionnaires were used to collect additional information about ease of use and comfort. Information regarding numbers of patients nursed on the mattresses during the trial period and details such as patient weight was not collected.

The results showed that none of the mattresses suffered from grounding and the two types of foam appeared to perform equally well. It was hoped to obtain some information regarding the effectiveness of the mattresses in preventing pressure ulcers, but as only one ward actually used the mattresses for patients at moderate risk of pressure ulcer development, the weekly audits were inconclusive.

Discussion

Once the bed was made, the Vaperm™ mattress could not easily be distinguished from the standard hospital mattresses, despite a small marker on the bed frame. The nurse questionnaires confirmed that the mattresses were satisfactory to use and easy to clean but it should be noted they were not, at that time, accustomed to think about the use of mattresses for pressure ulcer prevention. The patient questionnaires were not quantifiable as the patients' expectations of hospital mattresses were low and the most frequent comment was that the mattress was not bad – for a hospital mattress! Upon reflection, this study was over-ambitious in trying to measure efficacy of pressure ulcer prevention as well as the durability of the foam using inadequate methods. It was also noted that the wording in the evaluative questionnaires was poor, which also contributed to the unsatisfactory outcome.

Research lessons learned from this study

As a result of this experience a number of lessons were learned:

- The difficulty of keeping track of research equipment once it is placed in the clinical area. Clinical staff do not generally consider research equipment as different to any other equipment on the ward, for example the mattresses (and bed frame) were moved from ward to ward if the patient placed on it was transferred. This may be a particular problem if the research equipment is an everyday item such as a bed. This was evidenced by the fact that the nurses were often not aware that the mattress had actually gone to another ward.

• The study was undertaken in a 'real world' setting. That is, the mattresses were introduced as part of routine equipment. Education of the ward staff regarding the mattress usage, including discussion of the types of foam mattresses and their differences and the potential benefits for preventing pressure ulcers, might have impacted on the outcome of this small study. However, had this been done, different dimensions would have required evaluation. For example, was any positive outcome due to the mattress or to the increased knowledge base of nurses?

• Poor questionnaires yield poor data. Questionnaire development requires considerable skill. The author failed to take advantage of the many texts available on the subject and did not get advice from more experienced researchers. This was a particular problem at the time, as the locality in which the researcher worked did not have many support mechanisms for nurses new to research.

Exemplar 11.3

Background

The first prevalence survey of pressure ulcers undertaken in the elderly care hospital had revealed an overall prevalence rate of pressure sores in hospital patients of 33% (Dealey et al 1991). Of these, 38% were on the buttocks and 28% on the sacrum. As the majority of patients sat in the day room for most of the day, it was concluded that sitting rather than lying was a major factor in pressure ulcer development. A survey of the 119 armchairs for patient use revealed that only 28 (23%) were fit for purpose (Dealey et al 1991). The remaining chairs were in a poor state with damaged frame or coverings and/or grounding of the foam or indentation of the cushion. Little research was available in this area and an opportunity to undertake an evaluation of a relatively new chair with an integral pressure redistributing cushion was welcomed.

Method and results

A total of 22 patients at low to medium risk of pressure ulcer development used the chairs for a 1-week period. The patients had a nursing and physiotherapy assessment at the beginning and end of the week, which included skin status, level of mobility and a functional assessment for unsupported sitting. Interface pressure measurements at the ischial tuberosity were also taken, comparing a baseline measurement taken when the patient was seated on the canvas seat of a wheelchair to that when seated on the armchair.

The results demonstrated that the cushion provided adequate pressure relief for the patient group. Interface pressure measurements in the wheelchair ranged from 190 to 35 mmHg with there being considerable disparity between the pressures under each ischial tuberosity for nine patients. The most extreme example was one patient with a pressure of 110 mmHg under the right ischium and 35 mmHg under the left, indicating the patient tended to tilt sideways increasing the risk of pressure ulcer development on the right. In comparison, the interface pressure measurements in the armchair ranged from 18 to 60 mmHg and there was very little difference between pressure readings on the right and left sides which meant the patients were being supported in an upright position. However, the arms were too wide for people with small hands to grasp easily when rising to standing and were subsequently modified by the manufacturer. Although this may not appear to directly impact on pressure ulcer development, the problem was relevant as the wide arms impacted on the mobility of some patients.

Discussion

There were a number of limitations to the study, not least that no attempt was made to undertake a comparative study using a range of different chairs and cushions. This type of research can be useful as an exploratory pilot study in order to develop suitable test methods for a comparative study, but on its own does not determine efficacy of a product. However, given the baseline situation observed – namely poor seating overall – this study did raise awareness within the hospital of the need to provide suitable seating for this group of elderly patients and resulted in funds being made available to purchase more chairs. Consequently it did have an impact on service provision.

Another problem was the initial inadequacy of the physiotherapy assessment in relation to maintenance of posture. Initially data relating to any patient's tendency to fall backwards or forwards when sitting without support were not recorded. However, this was later rectified and the information was collected on all patients. Modification of data collection during a study is not good practice and reinforces the need for careful planning and an initial pilot study.

A major failing was the limited communication between the researchers and the ward staff. As patients were recruited to the study, one of the researchers explained the procedure to a senior nurse on the ward. Unfortunately this information was not always relayed to the other nurses on the ward and this sometimes led to loss of data. For example, one patient was discharged shortly before the researchers arrived to undertake the final measurements. It would have been unethical to delay the patient's discharge for research purposes, but if the ward staff had alerted the research team they would have visited the ward earlier to collect the final data.

Research lessons learned from this study

The lessons learned in this study were:

- The importance of undertaking a pilot study to test the data collection tool as discussed above.
- The need to ensure that *all* staff in the clinical area are aware if research is ongoing in the clinical areas. It is easy to make assumptions about the communication system within the clinical area and to forget the impact that factors

such as workload and shift patterns can have on any system, even those that are relatively effective.

 • Linked with this it is important to be alert to the fact that others will not be aware of the importance of your research. Many factors impact on this including education and research awareness (see Ch. 6), clinical workload, staffing issues, etc. Clinical colleagues will not automatically tell the rest of the team about your study; as a researcher, you have to do it yourself.

Exemplar 11.4

Background

The survey of armchairs within the elderly care hospital had identified that a number of chairs did not provide very good functional support for patients or provide pressure relief and were also in a poor state of repair with torn covers. Upon discussion with the ward staff it was discovered that these chairs were used for patients with considerable seating difficulties, such that they could not sit in an ordinary chair without sliding out. Some of these patients had contracted legs and several were confused or agitated, thus safety as well as positioning was a factor in their care. An alternative to these chairs was being sought when the author was approached with a request to evaluate a chair called the Fallout Chair™. This chair had been developed in Australia specifically for people with Huntington's disease and appeared to be a very suitable replacement chair. The aim of the study was to evaluate the Fallout Chair™ objectively to see if it resolved some of the specific problems associated with caring for patients with severe postural problems (Eden et al 1992).

Methods and results

A total of 18 patients were to be recruited to the study. Following an initial assessment, which included skin status at sacrum and buttocks, mental status, nursing problems and functional seating problems, each patient used a chair for a week. Interface pressure readings were also taken comparing a baseline of the patient sitting on the canvas seat of a wheelchair with the Fallout Chair™.

Although 18 patients were recruited to the study, two withdrew after a couple of days. Both these patients were younger disabled patients who decided that the chair was more suitable for 'old people'. The remaining patients had multiple pathologies and problems that made statistical analysis impossible. However, all the patients were at moderate to high risk of developing pressure ulcers and 10 of the 16 (62.5%) actually had pressure ulcers. Twelve patients (75%) had an initial problem of sliding out of conventional chairs. Eight of the patients (50%) were confused and/or agitated.

Twelve patients were found to have improvements in their specific problems following the use of the chair. Patients did not slide out of it and a very ill patient found it comfortable to sit out in for short periods. A number of patients who required feeding were fed while sitting in the chair and this identified a problem for one patient with a swallowing difficulty, in that the chair exacerbated the problem. The interface pressure measurements showed a reduction from the baseline for all but two patients with the interface pressures reduced from a range of 160–310 mmHg on the wheelchair canvas to less than 60 mmHg in the chair, a very satisfactory measurement in terms of pressure ulcer prevention. Both the patients whose interface pressures did not reduce significantly had had bilateral amputation of the legs. The interface pressure at the sacrum for one of the patients remained at 310 mmHg suggesting that the chair was not suitable for this group of patients. The ward nurses also reported that the confused patients were less agitated and did not shout as much as when seated in their usual chairs, although this was a subjective observation.

Discussion

The study demonstrated that the Fallout Chair™ was useful for a number of patients with complex seating difficulties. It was thought that the reason that so many of the confused patients seemed calmer was because they felt more comfortable and 'safer' in the Fallout Chair™ compared to their usual chair. This caused distress to many of the nurses that they had not recognized the true reason for agitation. However, this was only a subjective opinion and no formal assessment measures were used to measure distress levels. It must also be noted that this was a very small sample of patients and so no definitive conclusions can be drawn from the study.

Research lessons learned from this study

This study demonstrated the complexity of attempting an evaluation with a patient group that has diverse problems. Upon reflection some of these issues could have been addressed by more careful collection of data. For example, there are a variety of validated tools available to assess the mental status and stress levels of patients. Had greater detail been available on these aspects it might have enabled some stronger conclusions about the suitability of these chairs for patients with specific problems. Again it was noted that collaboration with experienced researchers would have resulted in more rigorous methods being implemented.

Exemplar 11.5

Background

Research does not occur in a vacuum. The early 1990s were a busy time for developments in pressure ulcer prevention strategies. A very important publication was *Pressure Sores: a Key Quality Indicator* (Department of Health 1993), which recognized that the incidence of pressure ulcers could be used to measure the quality of care provided within a healthcare setting. The previous year, the White

Paper *The Health of the Nation* (Department of Health 1992) had called for an annual reduction in pressure ulcer incidence of 5–10%. The use of pressure redistributing equipment was seen to be an important aspect of care. However, there was a lack of research to justify the use of many of the products (Young 1992, Bliss & Thomas 1993). Clark & Cullum (1992) had found that uncontrolled purchase of equipment was not the answer, as they found an increase in pressure ulcer prevalence despite an increase in the number of specialist mattresses.

Bliss & Thomas (1993) called for more randomized control trials of equipment to determine efficacy, but little funding was available at the time for large-scale studies. Most manufacturers were unwilling to expend the large sums of money required without some initial clinical evaluation. Others hoped that a simple evaluation would be sufficient. It was within this scenario that the Nimbus II™ dynamic flotation mattress was launched in 1993. It was an improved version of the original Nimbus™ mattress. The author was asked to participate in the initial clinical evaluation (Dealey 1994b). One potential benefit was being able to retain the mattresses for clinical use after the research, an aspect highlighted in Exemplar 11.2. Such benefits, however, need to be viewed with caution as there is the risk that offers of material benefits in research may be seen as a form of coercion. Furthermore, in the context of clinical governance (see Ch. 4) care must be taken to ensure that research related activities fit with managerial policies that govern procurement of equipment.

Methods and results

Four mattresses were supplied to the acute hospital and one placed in each of four different clinical areas: cardiac intensive care, renal surgery, neurology and care of the elderly. These areas were selected because the nurses were familiar with the original Nimbus™ mattress and were most likely to use it effectively and appropriately. Each ward was asked to monitor five patients over a 3-month period. Patients could be recruited if they were at medium to high risk of developing pressure ulcers using the Waterlow score. Training on the use of the mattress was provided by a company representative. The evaluation sought to measure the incidence of pressure ulcers, any improvement in existing pressure ulcers, ease of use and comfort. All pressure ulcers were measured for greatest length, greatest width and depth.

Fourteen patients with an age range of 26–87 years (mean 70 years) completed the evaluation. Seven of the patients had a total of 16 pressure ulcers. All were at moderate to high risk of pressure ulcer development.

In terms of outcomes, none of the patients developed pressure ulcers while on the mattress. Five of the seven patients with pressure ulcers showed an improvement in ulcers, either complete healing or a reduction in ulcer size as shown from the recorded measurements at the beginning and end of the evaluation. The remaining two patients subsequently died and their pressure ulcers may have been an indicator of the severity of their illness.

The evaluation showed that the nurses found the mattress easy to use. They particularly liked the transport facility (a switch on the mattress which ensured it remained inflated while the electrical supply was cut off for a short period). The transport facility was used for nine of the 14 patients as they were either moved within the ward or transferred to another ward. The nurses considered that the transport facility was an extremely useful benefit of the mattress. No problems were found when providing nursing care for patients.

Only eight patients were able to complete the patient evaluation forms; the other six were unable to do so because of their mental or physical condition. All the eight patients found the mattress comfortable and did not have any problems getting on or off the mattress.

Discussion

There were considerable problems collecting the data for this study. The nurses in the clinical areas were asked to identify suitable patients for the mattress and to complete the data collection forms. Some failed to do so adequately so that a number of forms had so little data that they were unusable at the analysis stage. Another problem was that the data collection forms tended to get mislaid, especially when a patient was transferred from one ward to another. Consequently in this research study, the CNS spent much time trying to track down forms and to get them completed. It appeared that although the nurses were keen to acquire the mattresses at the end of the study, they were not particularly interested in undertaking the data collection.

Research lessons learned from this study

This study demonstrated that completion of data collection forms was very low in the priorities of the ward nurses. It was recognized that high quality data may be best achieved by having a dedicated person to collect it. When there is one person whose key task is to recruit patients into a study and to complete all the relevant data collection forms there is a greater chance of ensuring that more patients are recruited to the study in the first instance and all relevant data is collected. This was, however, a challenging thought for the CNS who remained firmly committed to develop research in practice with practitioners. As demonstrated in Exemplar 11.1, there are some situations in which working with practitioners worked very well and facilitated the collection of large amounts of data. This would have been more difficult for a single researcher to do. Consequently it appears that each situation is different but must be very carefully thought through.

Exemplar 11.6

Background

After the problems in obtaining data in the previously described study, the author determined that all further studies would only be undertaken with the assistance of

Table 11.2 Clinical trial standards

- Appropriate research protocol developed to meet study aims
- Clear inclusion and exclusion criteria
- Measurable outcomes
- Local research ethics committee approval obtained
- Papers prepared for presentation at agreed conferences and publication in peer reviewed journals

a research nurse with specialist knowledge of tissue viability. This nurse would be able to identify suitable patients and recruit them to a relevant study. Such a post had to be financed by funds obtained for undertaking studies. The author was also influenced by a discussion paper by Cullum (1996), which emphasized the importance of having well constructed clinical trials. Cullum's check-list gave guidance to the paper prepared by the author to determine what she was able to offer to companies interested in sponsoring a clinical trial. Table 11.2 provides a synopsis of the paper.

Exemplar 11.6 is one of a number of studies undertaken at this time and involved an observational study of the Autoexcel™ mattress overlay (Keogh & Dealey 1997). The Autoexcel™ mattress overlay is an alternating air overlay with firm edges along its length, which provide support for patients when sitting on the side of the bed.

The study was an exploratory study to examine the feasibility of undertaking a randomized control trial if the results were promising. The aim of the study was to assess the effects of using the overlay for a group of elderly patients at high risk of pressure ulcer development in respect of pressure ulcer healing and prevention and patient and user acceptability.

Methods and results

The research nurse visited each ward in the elderly care hospital frequently to encourage staff to identify suitable patients. The range of inclusion and exclusion criteria was set based on the parameters of the mattress performance and ethical considerations. Thus, patients involved in the study needed to weigh between 45 and 203 kg to be included in the study. Those with mental frailty or a terminal illness were excluded. Thirty patients meeting the inclusion criteria were to be observed using the mattress overlay for a 3-week period. Their ages ranged from 49 to 94 years (mean 76 years) and their Waterlow risk scores ranged from 16 to 27 (median score was 21). Following initial assessment, each patient was assessed weekly for skin status and progress of existing pressure ulcers. A patient questionnaire and a nurse questionnaire were completed at the end of the study period.

Thirty patients entered the study but two had to be excluded from the analysis as only baseline data had been collected. Of these two, one patient died and the other had to be transferred to another mattress because of a minor fault in the trial mattress overlay. The results from the remaining 28 patients were analysed.

These patients remained in the trial for a mean of 19 days (range 7–21 days). Seven patients did not complete the 21 days because of: discharge/transfer (five patients), fall resulting in a fracture (one patient) and overlay uncomfortable (one patient).

None of the patients developed a pressure ulcer while on the overlay. Seventeen patients had existing pressure ulcers and seven of these patients had multiple ulcers – a total of 29 pressure ulcers. At the end of the study 17 (59%) had healed and a further 10 (34%) were improved.

Although the patients had a variety of diagnoses it was noted that 23 (79.3%) were in hospital for rehabilitation in order to maximize their physical abilities. For this reason, ease of movement both on the bed and in transferring from the bed was very important. The questionnaire for nurses explored whether patients were easy to reposition and transfer when using the mattress overlay. In 23 (79.3%) of cases the nurses agreed repositioning and transfer of patients was easy. The patients were not asked the same questions directly but several commented that they found independent transfers from bed to wheelchair easier than their previous overlay. Patients were asked about the comfort of the overlay. Data were missing for four patients; of the remaining 24 patients, 19 (79.2%) found the mattress to be comfortable or very comfortable. One patient found the mattress very uncomfortable and two found it uncomfortable. Eighteen patients of 24 (75%) (data missing for four patients) found that they had a good or very good night's sleep on the overlay.

Discussion

Having a dedicated research nurse to recruit patients and to collect the data made a considerable difference to the quality of the data collected. Moreover, lessons learned from previous work were well utilized, and more clearly defined outcome measures made the results easier to analyse. The study was a simple observational study and as such does not provide the level of confidence that can be obtained from a randomized control trial. However, it did indicate that the methods adopted would be suitable for a larger trial and so as a feasibility study this work achieved its purpose.

Research lessons learned from this study

As with the other studies, lessons were learned from this work.

- A dedicated person responsible for recruitment and data collection improves the quality of both recruitment and data. Patients were properly screened for suitability for the study ensuring that all possible patients were recruited. The data collection forms were completed correctly allowing for a more complete analysis than had been possible in some of the earlier studies.
- The need to grasp opportunities to learn from others. The author was able to learn from publications such as Cullum (1996) and to move forward in developing greater research skills and understanding. This was probably not uncommon at the time as many nurse researchers were looking to improve their skills.

- Increased awareness identified the need for a randomized control trial to demonstrate the efficacy of equipment. Use of randomization ensures that there is no difference between the control and experimental groups within a study, reducing the risk of both bias and chance affecting the results.

Exemplar 11.7

Background

The previous exemplars have demonstrated the progress made by the author in developing research skills. To some extent parallels can be drawn with the development of a more critical approach to research in tissue viability that Clark (1998) described as being in its infancy. A discussion of a review of 29 randomized control trials of pressure redistributing mattresses reported that the studies were generally of poor quality and the numbers were often too small to be of value (Cullum et al 1999). The author felt challenged to analyse her own research path (outlined above) and to utilize the learning noted in each exemplar. It was recognized that undertaking high-quality research could result in many challenges (Dealey 1998). Guidance was becoming more available to assist in achieving high standards from reports such as that by Prescott et al (1999). There are also guidelines such as the CONSORT (Consolidated Standards for Reporting Trials) statement (Moher et al 2001) to aid reporting clinical trials.

The chance to test these new insights into research methodology and put these resolves into practice came with a request to undertake a comparative study for a new electrically powered multi-sectioned profiling bed (Keogh & Dealey 2001). The aims of the study were to compare the use of electrically powered multi-sectioned profiling beds with a standard hospital bed with pressure relieving equipment for a group of patients at high risk of pressure ulcer development in respect of pressure ulcer incidence and patient handling and mobility.

Methods and results

The study was a randomized control trial. The control group was provided with a standard hospital bed plus an appropriate pressure relieving mattress and the experimental group provided with an electrically powered multi-sectioned profiling bed. Pressure relieving equipment for the control group was chosen based on existing hospital policy which indicated specific types of pressure redistributing equipment according to the patient's level of risk of pressure ulcer development. The experimental group had a pressure reducing foam mattress.

A power calculation (a statistical means of determining if the sample size is adequate to achieve a significant result for a given population) was undertaken and determined that 450 patients in each arm of the study would need to be recruited to achieve the main aim of the study; far smaller numbers were required to achieve a significant result for the secondary aims. A block design, computer generated code was provided by an independent statistician. An assistant placed the allocation for each patient into sealed opaque envelopes that were numbered sequentially. Thus, neither the clinical investigator nor the patient knew the bed allocation until after recruitment.

Patients were selected according to a strict inclusion/exclusion criteria and participated in the study for a minimum of 5 days and a maximum of 10 days. Initial demographic data were collected and patients were assessed for skin status and pressure ulcer risk daily. At the end of the study each patient was given a questionnaire to complete regarding mobility while on the bed and during transfers from the bed. A total of 100 nurses were given a semi-structured questionnaire asking them to compare the two bed types. In addition, case studies were undertaken of six patients who were placed on the trial bed by ward nurses in the absence of the clinical investigator. None of these patients met the inclusion criteria for the study but they were too ill to be transferred to another bed.

A total of 100 patients were recruited in the time available. Data were incomplete for 30 patients, but all 100 patients were included in the intent-to-treat analysis of the primary outcome of pressure ulcer incidence. There was an incidence of 0% in both groups. The 30 patients with incomplete data were excluded from the analysis of the secondary outcome measures.

In summary, there were 35 patients in each group whose results were analysed. The demographic details for each group revealed that they were comparable groups. There was a significant difference between the two groups of patients in favour of the experimental bed in respect of the ease of change of position in bed ($p = 0.0014$); maintaining a sitting balance ($p = 0.001$) and transferring from the bed ($p = 0.0001$). The nurses' survey had a 75% ($n = 75$) response rate and reflected the views of 62.5% of the nurses from the six wards participating in the study. Again there was a significant response to the experimental bed in respect of ease of undertaking nursing duties ($p = 0.0001$); repositioning of patients ($p = 0.0033$); patients being able to reposition themselves ($p = 0.0001$). Seventy-four (98.67%) of the nurses stated that they would use the experimental bed to care for heavily dependent, immobile patients. This statement was supported by the type of patients in the case studies, all of whom fell into this category. It should also be noted that all of these patients were at very high risk of pressure ulcer development, but none of this group developed pressure ulcers.

Discussion

Obviously the numbers of patients recruited fell far short of the numbers indicated by the power calculation. This was in part because of over-optimism of the researchers of the numbers of available patients and the numbers that it was feasible to have in the study at any one time. Also the system of allocating patients to groups did not work at weekends when the research nurse was not available. However, the highly significant results in relation to patient movement in the bed and for transfers has the potential to impact on friction and shear, both factors in pressure ulcer development.

Ideally, this type of study should also include an economic analysis such as a cost-benefit analysis. Unfortunately there was insufficient funding to permit this to be included in the study. Realistically, recruitment of such large numbers as were required for this study can only be achieved by means of a multi-centre study (see Ch. 12). This type of study is extremely expensive and can probably only be achieved by obtaining an externally funded, non-commercial research grant. Unfortunately, the challenges of obtaining research funding pertain to this type of work as well as others (see Ch. 2).

It must also be noted that the case studies were an add-on to the study to try and obtain a clearer picture of the type of patient that the nurses deemed required the electrically operated beds. It is not good practice to change study methods part-way through a study. These case studies did not represent a change in methods, more the collection of information to clarify some of the problems in recruitment.

Research lessons learned from this study

The learning continued with this study and it was noted:

- It is unrealistic to expect to recruit large numbers of patients from one centre. Most research is time-limited and therefore there needs to be a steady flow of patient recruitment. It is difficult for one research nurse to screen large numbers of patients and recruit and maintain data collection, particularly in a study that required the movement of beds and often the delivery of a bed to the ward from the equipment store.

- However well devised, ward nurses will circumvent clinical trial methods if they believe it is in the best interest of their patients. Despite the education provided by the research nurse which was reinforced by both written material and notices on the wards, in the absence of the research nurse, the ward nurses utilized the electric beds as they believed best, regardless of the study. This demonstrates the ongoing challenge to increase the research awareness of clinical staff (see Ch. 4). While doing what they felt 'best', the nurses lack of knowledge of the outcome of the research must be acknowledged and that there is an ongoing need to instil an evidence-based culture without alienating clinical staff.

- Another interesting lesson from this study was related to the costs of using new equipment. Although the electric profiling beds were supplied by the manufacturer for use in the study there was limited storage space in the hospital for displaced beds. This resulted in further costs as the displaced beds had to be placed in rented storage. No additional costs were required for the patients in the control group as they were placed on existing equipment stock.

- The recognition of the importance of economic evaluations of new equipment has developed over recent years. Within the world of healthcare there will always be limited or competing demands and so economic evaluation will add weight to the best use of limited resources. This type of evaluation is complex as it can involve measuring a mixture of depreciation of existing stock, purchase of new stock and some rental of equipment. The support of a health economist is required to ensure robust methods are used. Consequently, such studies will be more costly to undertake and need to be funded by research grants.

OTHER ISSUES TO CONSIDER IN RESEARCH

Ethical issues

Over the last 10 years or so there has rightly been increasing attention on the ethical issues surrounding medical research (see Ch. 12). The studies described within the exemplars need to be seen in the light of the time when they were undertaken. For example, regulations concerning research ethics have changed considerably since 1990/1 when Exemplar 11.4 was undertaken. Consultation with the chairman of the local research ethics committee at the time had confirmed that ethical approval was not necessary for an evaluation of this type of equipment. Thus, consent forms were not required to be completed by the participants. A full explanation and an invitation to participate were given to those patients who could understand. The confused patients were given a simple explanation and included in the study. This would be deemed unethical today, especially as several had no family to give assent to participation in the study. The dilemma is that this group of patients particularly benefited from the chair, a fact that might not have been uncovered but for this research.

Funding for research

The studies described within the exemplars were either funded in-house – that is, undertaken as part of day to day work of the CNS and other staff – or commercially funded. There are obvious limitations in commercially funded studies in that there is the risk that a company may try to influence the reporting of the results or selectively use some of the results in advertising material. Against this, there is the obvious advantage of being able to obtain much needed equipment for which there is no available funding within a hospital budget. It should also be noted that most commercial companies now adhere to the European Union *Good Clinical Practice Guidelines* for research which ensures that studies are conducted to a high standard (European Union 1996). When conducting any commercially funded research it is advisable to have a written agreement or contract regarding the terms of a study in advance. All such contracts should be overlooked by someone with knowledge of this type of documentation and signed by a senior member of staff who has the authority so to do, within the healthcare setting (see Ch. 2).

A more ideal method of funding is that obtained from research grants. There are a wide variety of bodies that provide research grants, generally on an annual basis. Many of these awards are considered to be highly prestigious.

Unsurprisingly, there is considerable competition for these monies and an expectation that applicants will comprise a team of academics and clinicians with a proven track record in research. There is no place for the lone researcher in this arena. Reaching this point of understanding has been an important step in my research journey. Like many other nurses, I have been guilty of undertaking poor quality research and failing to understand the importance of working within a multi-professional research team. Nurses often believe that they fail to receive research grants because funding bodies do not understand 'nursing research'; the reality may be that the quality of the proposed study is not of sufficiently high standard. This has been well evidenced in the personal research journey highlighted above which has tracked developments from naïve enthusiasm to tightly managed research. Parallels can be drawn with this research experience and the increased knowledge of developing research in healthcare today (see Ch. 6).

SUMMARY AND CONCLUSION

This chapter has sought to demonstrate the journey of one individual both in undertaking research to resolve clinical questions and developing research skills. This journey reflects the progress in research undertaken in tissue viability generally and also developments within the nursing profession in relation to research. It is important that this chapter is understood within the context of the time period in which it is set.

The conclusions that can be drawn are as follows:

- Novice researchers need to recognize their limitations and seek assistance from more experienced researchers, ideally within a research team
- All research studies should be adequately planned with a protocol outlining clear outcomes, inclusion and exclusion criteria, the use of validated assessments whenever possible and a pilot study to test the proposed methods
- The use of dedicated researchers to collect data ensures reliable outcomes
- The purpose of clinical research is to gain a better understanding of the impact of disease and how it might be prevented or treated. Clinical staff cannot divorce themselves from research as they should be involved in setting the research agenda, even if they do not directly participate in research studies.

REFERENCES

Bliss M R, Thomas J M 1993 Clinical trials with budgetry implications: establishing randomised trials of pressure relieving aids. Professional Nurse 8(5): 292–296
Bours G, Halfens R J, Lubbers M, Haalboom J R 1999 The development of a national registration form to measure the prevalence of pressure ulcers in the Netherlands. Ostomy and Wound Management 45(11): 28–33

Clark M 1998 Removing the 'estimates and guesses' from practice – evidence based tissue viability. Journal of Tissue Viability 8(2): 3–5

Clark M, Cullum N 1992 Matching patient need for pressure sore prevention with the supply of pressure redistributing mattresses. Journal of Advanced Nursing 17: 310–316

Cullum N 1996 Evaluation of treatments for wounds in clinical trials. Journal of Wound Care 5(1): 8–9

Cullum N, Deeks J, Sheldon T A, Song F, Fletcher A W 1999 Beds, mattresses and cushions for pressure sore prevention and treatment. In: Cochrane Library. Update Software, Oxford, issue 3

Dealey C 1988 The role of the tissue viability nurse. Nursing Standard 10(4): 16–19

Dealey C 1991 The size of the pressure sore problem in a teaching hospital. Journal of Advanced Nursing 16: 663–670

Dealey C 1992 A comparative study of two types of foam within Vaperm mattresses. Journal of Tissue Viability 2(2): 69–70

Dealey C 1994a Monitoring the pressure sore problem in a teaching hospital. Journal of Advanced Nursing 20: 652–659

Dealey C 1994b Evaluation of the Nimbus II mattress. Professional Nurse 9(12): 789–804

Dealey C 1997 Managing pressure sore prevention. Mark Allen Publishing, Salisbury

Dealey C 1998 Obtaining the evidence for clinically effective wound care. British Journal of Nursing 7(20): 1236–1240

Dealey C 2000 Pressure ulcer prevention strategies – are the data valid? Journal of Wound Care 9(7): 326

Dealey C, Earwaker T, Eden L 1991 Are your patients sitting comfortably. Journal of Tissue Viability 1(2): 36–39

Department of Health 1992 The health of the nation. HMSO, London

Department of Health 1993 Pressure sores: a key quality indicator. Department of Health, London

Eden L, Earwaker T, Dealey C 1992 The management of patients with major seating difficulties. In: Harding K G, Leaper D L, Turner T D (eds) Proceedings of the 1st European Conference on Advances in Wound Management. Macmillan Magazines, London

European Union 1996 Guidance on good clinical practice (CPMP/ICH/135/95). European Union, Brussels

Keogh A, Dealey C 1997 An observational study of the Autoexcel mattress overlay. In: Leaper D J, Cherry C W, Dealey C, Lawrence J C, Turner T D (eds) Proceedings of the 6th European Conference on Advances in Wound Care. Macmillan Magazines, London

Keogh A, Dealey C 2001 Profiling beds versus standard hospital beds: effects on pressure ulcer incidence outcomes. Journal of Wound Care 10(2): 15–19

Lowthian P 1989 Pressure sore prevention. Nursing 3: 17–23

Moher D, Schultz K F, Altman D 2001 The CONSORT statement: revised recommendations for improving the quality of reports of parallel-group randomised trials. Lancet 357: 1191–1194

Prescott R J, Counsell C E, Gillespie W J et al 1999 Factors that limit the quality, number and progress of randomised controlled trials. Health Technology Assessment 3(20): 1–151

Scales J T, Lowthian P T, Poole A G, Ludman W R 1982 Vaperm patient support system: a new general purpose hospital mattress. Lancet 20: 1150–1152

Waterlow J 1985 A risk assessment card. Nursing Times 81(48): 49–55

Young J 1992 The use of specialised beds and mattresses. Journal of Tissue Viability 2(3): 79–81

Implications

PART CONTENT

Research and development in practice

Collette Clifford

INTRODUCTION

In this chapter we will examine the wide-ranging issues that have emerged in the earlier chapters and consider the implications for the future management of research activity from both a research and development (R&D) perspective. In so doing we will focus on research as a medium for expansion of knowledge, and development as the utilization of knowledge generated by research in practice.

If we were to put some kind of measure in terms of healthcare staff involvement with R&D, undoubtedly it is the development aspect that would gain the greater weighting. The use of knowledge generated by research is the aspect that should be of interest to most healthcare practitioners because, in healthcare today, using research is not an optional extra, rather it is an integral part of professional practice. All healthcare practitioners should be able to give an account of the extent to which their practices have been informed by the best knowledge available. The purpose of research is to generate the 'best knowledge'; however, in order to generate this we need skilled researchers who will spend most of their working life in a research role. To develop this group we need to think of appropriate career paths coupled with the opportunity to develop the skills required to become researchers.

One way of considering how health professionals can be involved in research is to refer to the diagram in Figure 12.1. Here three broad areas of activity are identified: using research, participating in research and leading research.

Using research

The base of the triangle in Figure 12.1 represents the majority of the healthcare workforce. It would not be a realistic proposition to suggest that all should be involved in carrying out research but in present day healthcare it is important that all healthcare practitioners use relevant research as appropriate in their practice. This is no longer an optional extra and now forms a key aspect of research governance in healthcare in the NHS as documented in the Department of Health guidelines for research governance that can be found on the department's website (http://www.doh.gov.uk). We are in

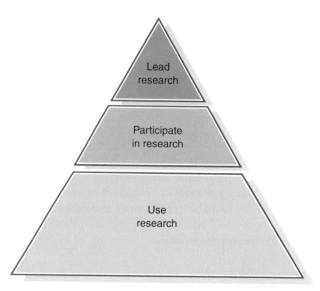

Figure 12.1 Level of research involvement.

a world in which information is readily available to anyone who has access to internet facilities. More and more people have this resource in their own homes and, if not, they can go to public libraries and access internet material that way. We only need to turn the clock back 15–20 years to understand what a radical change this is, a change that has impacted on the lives of millions of people – ready access to information on a wide range of subjects as and when required. The implications for health are that the general public now have access to the most up-to-date research information at the same time as the healthcare professionals (see Ch. 2). This means that the knowledge base of patients and clients using healthcare services are radically different to those of their predecessors who tended to look to professional groups as the main source of information and advice. We now live in a very different society in which the role of the user, a well informed user more often than not, is at the heart of healthcare. Consequently it is essential that healthcare professionals are 'on top' of the knowledge base relevant to their practice. The health professional role is changing from a paternalistic one in which the doctor, nurse or therapist advises the patient or client which treatment they think the best (often those based on custom and practice) to one in which the health professional lays the best knowledge in front of the patient or client and discusses the treatment options with them. Health professionals can only do this if they have the necessary information to do so and practice their work in a way in which research is utilized.

While this may be seen as a good standard of practice, efforts to get to this level of research utilization are not without challenge. As seen in several chapters (Chs 6, 7, 8 and 9) in this book, the starting point for a number of contributors was to identify what staff working in clinical units, the front line of healthcare, knew about research. It is not possible for staff to use research if their understanding of the processes involved and their ability to make judgements upon research outcomes is limited. It is clear from some of the reports here that much work still needs to be done to help those staff who have not had opportunity to develop their understanding of research and using research in practice.

Linked with this, there is clear recognition that even if the workforce had this level of understanding it would not be sensible for numerous different individuals to spend a lot of time undertaking systematic reviews of research evidence relevant to their area of practice each time they wanted to review how best to give care. Hence, as noted in Chapters 2, 3 and 4, the evolution of systematic review programmes completed by centres such as the Cochrane Centre was one clear way of helping hard-pressed practitioners get ready access to the most up-to-date and collective research findings related to their area of practice. This is one way of trying to circumvent a major replication of workload and make life easier for those working in practice. As centres established to undertake systematic reviews have evolved and increased their contribution to disseminating research findings then, accordingly, so their accessibility through web-based systems has developed (see, for example, http://www.cochrane.co.uk and http://www.jr2.ox.ac.uk/bandolier).

While the mechanisms to improve dissemination of research activity to help practitioners increase the use of research in practice have been developed it is worth noting that, in the best research tradition, the outcomes of recommendations from research reviews are also open to challenge. The ideology behind the service provided by, for example, the National Institute for Clinical Excellence (NICE) is one which blends the key aspects of evidence-based practice – i.e. research evidence – with, in the absence of research knowledge, the best available evidence. In critiquing findings experts may differ in their interpretations. Moreover, as indicated in earlier chapters, within publicly funded healthcare settings, research evidence is commonly considered alongside economic considerations, a factor that can lead to challenges in decision-making. A well informed public may accept that a particular approach to care is costly but they may not accept that this should be a reason for withholding the treatment if they require it. Years ago such debates would not have been raised in the public domain as health service management was a much more opaque process than it is today. To ensure greater transparency, even those who undertake tasks involved in reviewing healthcare research have said they should themselves come under critical scrutiny about the ways in which they undertake the processes. It is for this reason that, in 2003, NICE itself invited closer scrutiny of the way in which the institute's work is undertaken and it announced it will now be audited by the World Health Organization (WHO) (see http://www.nice.org.uk).

From another perspective, while such developments are commendable, it should be recognized that research knowledge development is a slow process. Associated with this, work undertaken to provide systematic reviews of practice will be constrained by the research knowledge available for review. For many aspects of healthcare this remains the challenge and so when discussions are undertaken with regard to 'getting research into practice', it must be acknowledged that a range of factors will impact upon the individual ability to do so. If, as is demonstrated in Chapter 6, some health-care professional groups have only a relatively recent history of research activity, it is evident that it will take time to build up the research knowledge base for that aspect of practice. If there is little or no research 'output' the potential to undertake real critical appraisal of the research through systematic reviews will be curtailed.

So, from the perspective of using research in practice, while it is recognized that all healthcare practitioners need a basic understanding of research processes to be able to use research outcomes in their work, this alone is not enough. Research needs to be available and there need to be good systems to help practitioners determine the quality of that research. As demonstrated in the various reports in this text, there is a lot of work to do to help nurture questioning and reflective approaches to work at an individual healthcare practitioner level. This is critical if we are to reach the ideology that all health-care practitioners will be using research in practice. Coupled with this, at an organizational level, it is necessary to ensure that managerial practice supports critical and reflective approaches to work and that those who are willing to do this work do not themselves become static in healthcare delivery.

Participating in research

The next part of the triangle (Fig. 12.1) refers to participating in research. This has been highlighted to illustrate that a number of healthcare staff may, at various points in their career, have the opportunity to move beyond the theoretical base of what research is about and to take part in some aspects of the research process, participating in generating knowledge. This may include design and development of small-scale projects, perhaps as part of initial professional education (see Chs 6 and 7) or a course of study about research as part of continuing professional development (CPD). An increasing number of practitioners across a range of healthcare disciplines are choosing to undertake higher degrees that carry a specific research component. These range from masters degrees through to doctoral level study. Another group choose to undertake roles that offer substantive employment in undertaking a research project. For some, this experience may spark a lifelong interest in research and lead, at one level, to confidence in an approach to practice that ensures consistent use of 'best available knowledge'. For others the impact may vary as some, for example, choose to specialize in research work but may spend time in a research assistant role, supporting lead researchers in aspects of data collection. Should members of this group move to alternative employment at a later date their experience would give them the knowledge base essential to enable them to use research, as appropriate, in their work. At another level a number of healthcare staff use the opportunities created by participating in research, either as project team members or by undertaking further study, as a stepping-stone to a substantive research role and a career as a research leader.

Leading research

Differentiating the roles above is useful for it might be argued that each stage requires different knowledge and skill. Associated with this, as healthcare professionals have understood the process of managing research practices more fully, so the ways in which efforts have been made to support R&D activity have changed. Hence we saw the shift from the concept of 'getting research into practice' to the 'evidence-based practice' approach (see Ch. 2). Those staff who lead the research agenda need to understand the global picture about R&D and be able to support developments at each step of the process. As indicated in Chapter 2, at the beginning of the 21st century we have a much clearer picture of optimal ways and means of managing research than we had in the last decade of the 20th century.

Learning how best to lead a research agenda is another dimension worthy of exploration. It is worth reiterating the relatively short time-span over which many professional groups in healthcare have been learning about research. Contributors to this book have given accounts of their personal experiences of trying to help colleagues understand what it means to use research in practice and a number of organizational efforts have been cited. Less evident in this book is the teaching activity that occurs across the education sector as healthcare educators try to help newcomers to research learn about the research processes. For many this begins with learning how to critique research articles. In the 21st century such efforts form the first step in understanding the processes of systematic review. This can be compared with teaching models in the latter part of the 20th century in which students were commonly asked to read a research article and consider how the findings might impact on their practice. As the art of 'systematic reviews' of research studies became more established in healthcare it became apparent that only very rarely would there be enough evidence from a single piece of research work to recommend major changes in practice. This represents a shifting paradigm in the way in which research outputs were viewed by those in healthcare.

Other models have been used to try and develop research leaders, albeit at a local level. For example, exploration of ways of getting research into practice led to participatory models in which it was hoped that research leaders would arise from practice if given the opportunity to participate and lead their own research projects in clinical practice under close supervision. The conclusion of one study was that such models are not feasible unless there is full organizational commitment to supporting the research agenda, an aspect that did not develop in the locality where this project was undertaken due to major organizational change during the time span of the project (Clifford & Murray 2001). As indicated above, sometimes experience of research participation, at whatever level, does result in individual staff members developing greater understanding of research and subsequently taking on leadership roles. However, there remains, in many professional groups, a need to consider further how best to develop the next generation of research leaders. It is perhaps fair to say that visions of research leadership have undergone a change as for some the 'traditional' model of leading research project pertains, while for others leadership in research will focus on the development end, the use of research evidence in practice.

There is still a lot of work that needs to be undertaken to determine how best to develop leaders for research, particularly in those disciplines that do not have a long history in research development (HEFCE 2001).

The challenge of how best to develop research leaders is perhaps complicated by lack of clear answers to the simple question 'how many leaders are required for research?' This is not an easy question to answer as needs may vary by professional group, organizational structure, and aspects of care that need to be developed. The knowledge gained by all those contributing their efforts to this agenda can be seen in Chapters 6 to 11 but there are no clear answers as to the best way to lead research endeavours as the endeavours are themselves variable, crossing the boundaries between doing research and using research in practice.

Linked with this is the need, at one level, to identify sufficient finance to support the training and development of research leaders and at another to find ways of funding the research that is deemed appropriate for healthcare today (see Chs 2 and 3). The account in Chapter 11 of a personal journey through research illustrates the strong driving force that some individuals have to take a lead role in research. As a historical snapshot it is worth reviewing the experiences outlined in Chapter 11 alongside the time-scales of development of the R&D agenda in Chapters 2 and 3 and the educational development noted in Chapters 6 and 7. Here it can be seen that the evolution of support systems began to influence the way in which Dealey was able to approach her work in research in tissue viability. It is to be hoped that the systems established at the beginning of the 21st century will serve to give better support to the development of the next generation of researchers (see HEFCE 2001).

CONCLUSIONS

In Chapter 1 we presented a framework to set the scene for the broad context of this text (see Fig. 1.1, Ch. 1). This framework will underpin the following concluding sections as we address issues related to healthcare policy, education, knowledge and dissemination. The implications of some of the issues raised in this text will also be considered from the context of how best to ensure that research generated is utilized in healthcare practice today, in other words the implications for 'getting research into practice'.

HEALTHCARE RESEARCH POLICY

The future healthcare research policy relating to R&D in England will almost certainly continue to involve central government control, albeit with devolved responsibility to local clinical units, and with endeavours to ensure that the general public play a part in the evolving research agenda.

The early chapters in this book set out the changing face of health service research in one country. Here the shift was from research programmes inspired predominantly by individual interest to one which clearly focuses on health funded research into areas reflecting specific government targets for health. The success of this policy initiative is evident in a range of readily accessible healthcare research resources that can be accessed via the Department of Health website (http://www.doh.gov.uk). This includes not only a range of policy aspects related to R&D in healthcare in England but also the outcomes of that research. So, for example, the National Research Register (NRR 2003) gives full listings of health services-funded research and opens a forum by which researchers can readily communicate with each other. NICE (http://www.nice.org.uk) takes the evidence provided and, after full review, offers guidance to practitioners for a range of healthcare situations. While these are relatively new systems and, as noted above, not without challenge, there is little doubt they are making inroads into providing the best available evidence about specific lines of treatment to healthcare professionals.

Strategic management of dissemination and evidence-based practice

The health policy for R&D offers a 'total package' from inception of research ideas through to the dissemination of findings with a target to increase the use of research evidence in practice. From a policy perspective it should be noted that continued development of systematic reviews of existing research, sponsoring original research where necessary, and making research findings easily accessible nationally through readily accessible electronic databases have meant that much of the early vision of the NHS R&D strategy has been realized. At a national, strategic level, healthcare managers can point to the very obvious achievements in disseminating research and contributing to the development of a professional population that bases practice upon the evidence available.

Managerial accountability

A key component of the drive to integrate research into health policy is the introduction of systems of managerial accountability for research activity undertaken in the NHS. In the last 10 years new managerial systems for research have been developed at a local level. Not so many years ago such systems were non-existent and funding was simply allocated in an ad hoc way to teaching hospitals (see Ch. 2). In the early years of the 21st century there is increased recognition of the importance of developing research and an evidence-based culture within an environment in which consideration must be given to health economics and the cost-effectiveness of differing health technologies (see Ch. 3). This must be seen as a success story in terms of the changes made to the economic management of health services research. Having said that, it is worth noting that for many researchers the introduction of such systems has required a major culture change in their approach to research. Of necessity, new managerial systems and associated accountability have introduced new requirements into research work and brought additional workloads to healthcare organizations that have an active research profile. For those that do not get too involved in direct research activity managerial accountability for research remains but is focused on the evidence-based practice agenda.

At the level of 'doing research' these systems are now established through local R&D managers (see Ch. 2) but, as can be seen by several examples in this book, the challenge of finding ways of helping staff to find ways of using research in practice still remains. This is particularly challenging for the reasons noted above in that in healthcare today we expect that all care should be based upon best available knowledge.

Research governance

The concept of research governance reflects the managerial model of clinical governance that now underpins health services management in England (see Ch. 4). This offers a refinement of early systems designed to ensure that there is full accountability for research activity in NHS healthcare settings (http://www.doh.gov.uk). The research governance framework (Department of Health 2001) notes that it 'is essential that existing sources of evidence, especially systematic reviews, are considered carefully prior to undertaking research. Research which duplicates other work unnecessarily or which is not of sufficient quality to contribute something useful to existing knowledge is in itself unethical.' From this starting point the research governance framework sets standards for the overall management of research from the initial activity cited above to the financial and personal managerial issues related to research. This includes the need to have mechanisms by which clinical staff are fully informed of the research governance framework and the need to utilize an evidence-based agenda in healthcare. The challenges of achieving these targets are evidenced in the case study chapters presented here where it is apparent that there is much work to be done at practice level to support staff wishing to be confident of their ability to use research in practice (see Chs 6–11). Although the case studies presented were undertaken before the NHS research governance agenda was introduced they are an indicator of the nature of the challenge to health service managers who will need to be able to state with confidence that their staff are taking an evidence-based approach to their work.

Monitoring research from an ethical perspective

One aspect that has been referred to only briefly in some chapters in the book is that of ethics in research. However, given the increasing recognition of the importance of this (noted in Ch. 2), a short section has been included under research management as it is predicted that these systems will become more refined in the years ahead. Clearly there is a need for ethical issues to be managed separately from a strategy designed to promote research activity and to ensure that there are separate mechanisms for objective review of research being undertaken in healthcare settings. Systems for ethical review of research have been in existence for many years in the UK. Recently these have come under critical scrutiny both to ensure that practices are taking account of the changing face of health service research and to meet the standards required in all health services research, namely that the processes involved should be transparent and open. As a result a new organization has been developed within the Department of Health, the Central Office for Research Ethics Committees (http://www.corec.org.uk). This office has been given the remit of introducing governance arrangements into the management of ethics committees. This is an important development for the management of ethics committees, which in the past were very much left to local systems development. With the best will in the world, lack of central control of how the ethical dimension of research at local level was managed led to major challenges to researchers who felt they were working to different agendas depending upon the local research ethics committees they were dealing with. Hence the increased standardization of ethical systems is welcomed by most. Linked with this is the increased impact of the active participation of the UK within the European Union (EU). This means that from 2004 the systems for regulating ethics committees will extend beyond national guidelines as the EU requirements for ethical approval of clinical trials is introduced (European Union 2001). It is likely that the standards set for managing clinical trials will be applied to all other research activity in healthcare.

Consumer involvement

Another key challenge for healthcare research managers and researchers is how to ensure healthcare consumers are best involved in research (Department of Health 1999). This reflects an important shift in attitude in which those people who may volunteer to be involved in research do so as informed participants. The word 'subjects' commonly used in research textbooks when referring to the sample in research studies involving humans, has, for many people, become unacceptable: the term implies a passive stance in those people who are in fact contributing to the research in a most positive way in exposing themselves to perhaps new treatments or variations on treatment. As can be seen in Chapter 10, even for a small-scale pilot project this requires a lot of cooperation from patients using services and so it is only right and proper that they are fully informed as to what participation in research requires.

Space does not allow a full analysis of user involvement in research here although key issues are raised in Chapter 2. Suffice it to say that, as with other aspects of research development, a major philosophical shift can be seen in working towards a research agenda with full participative involvement of those people who will be the recipients of the research outcomes. Those who have always worked to high standards in ensuring full informed consent in research activity will say this has always been the case but sadly, as indicated in Chapter 2, evidence in recent years has indicated that this has not been so for all (Wilmshurst 2002). Moreover, even for those who have practised to optimal level it has not always been the norm to consider ways of involving consumers in research design and research management as part of the research governance directives.

EDUCATION

The second strand identified in the opening chapter was the importance of ensuring that education for healthcare professionals meets the demand for developing an evidence-based agenda in healthcare. The challenges posed in changing education provision in a relatively short time span are outlined in Chapter 6. Here the need to undertake parallel education of new students to the profession at the same time as lecturers was discussed. Similar challenges emerged in Chapter 7 and, as has been noted earlier, with the exception of the small number of professional groups that have always been educated in the university sector, the challenges of such parallel developments remains for all healthcare groups.

Future professional education will almost certainly continue to embrace ways of enhancing research development. However, there remain a number of issues that require further clarification to ensure that R&D in healthcare is at an optimal level.

The first issue is to consider what the optimal education package for future healthcare professionals comprises. At one level it may be suggested that this has developed in a very piecemeal way with a tendency for some programmes to concentrate on teaching people how to do research while others have, in more recent times, focused on the use of research, i.e. the evidence-based practice (EBP) agenda (see Ch. 2).

Linked with this has been the fact that healthcare education was formerly very much a unidisciplinary enterprise. One of the areas of interest arising out of current healthcare policy is an increased interest in learning and working together. This has evolved specifically out of the *NHS Plan* (Department of Health 2000) in which the focus on the needs of the consumer has raised questions about the tendency to define care by professional boundaries of activity. This is no longer seen as acceptable and so there are a number of initiatives designed to address the development needs to foster new ways of working in healthcare.

This needs to be considered from the perspective of research. It should be noted, however, that little is known about the 'best' way to do this. Evidence to date suggests that models of learning about research do differ across professional groups and that this may have an impact on the extent to which professional groups are prepared to use research in practice (Clifford et al 2002). However, greater understanding is required to support this agenda. In summary, there is a need for continued development of research knowledge and skills in pre- and post-registration education in all professional groups and, following on from this, continued development of multi-professional learning in pre- and post-registration programmes that fosters shared research initiatives.

To support such developments we need to continue building upon existing strengths in the development of university and service partnerships to support the educational agenda to underpin the use of research in practice.

EXISTING KNOWLEDGE, CUSTOMS AND PRACTICES

Chapters 4 and 5 outlined the complexities of introducing change into healthcare organizations. It must be acknowledged that if the agenda to ensure that healthcare practice is based on research is to move forward, healthcare organizations need to consider how they can create a research culture that fosters questioning, encourages change, and embraces the ethos of a learning organization. To achieve this there is a need for supportive strategic management that actively leads and resources a clear R&D strategy. This requires the active implementation of a philosophy that engenders an awareness of research in all staff which is reflected in job descriptions, CPD, individual performance review (IPR) and clinical supervision. This, as indicated in Chapter 4, is easier said than done but if the points above are considered from the perspective of the strategic requirement of the research governance agenda it can be seen that it is not impossible. However, managers need to consider the power of customs and practices in healthcare delivery and have clear strategies to help staff who might need to work in new ways.

DISSEMINATION

In order for the EBP agenda to move forward in the future, healthcare organizations need to consider the best ways of establishing improved dissemination and communication frameworks that include a dynamic database of staff research activity. This is important, for it is interesting to note that the vast amount of work undertaken at national level is not filtering through at the desired rate to people in practice. If it were, the reports here of efforts to 'get research into practice' would have met with much more positive outcomes and indeed little would remain to be done today.

Ways of doing this may include improved multi-professional networking that fosters sharing and provides peer support. The provision of more time for staff reflection and debate is an ideology that sadly cannot always be met in busy healthcare environments and lack of time is still often cited as the prime reason for the failure of staff to facilitate a research agenda. Aside from the experiences shared in this book there is ongoing and continuing evidence of struggles to get staff involved in research activity (Wye & McClenahan 2000, Thompson et al 2002, Bryar et al 2003).

When considering dissemination it is also important to make the links to the consumer view. Linked with this is the creation of a better awareness in healthcare professionals of the patient as an informed partner in all R&D activity. There is a lot of scope here to develop creative ways of dissemination that will help develop partnerships in the utilization of research in healthcare.

Enhanced provision of information technology (IT) at grass roots level that facilitates user-friendly access to electronic databases at point of need to all levels of healthcare professional is part of the government plan (Department of Health 2000). However, as with any major change, there is commonly a gap between the ideal and reality. There was a 'blip' in the early 1990s as a result of changes in healthcare education when resources that were tied up with educational funding were redirected to the university sector. This included library and IT facilities (see Ch. 2). This has been addressed and most NHS settings in England now have identifiable library resources for staff. The challenge is for staff to make time to access available resources. Although computers are being made more available to practitioners it is still not the norm for all healthcare practitioners to have ready, daily access to IT. Until this government target is achieved the R&D strategic developments will remain limited.

The final point in dissemination is a need to consider how best to create the culture that will encourage staff to make time to review and discuss the implication of research made available to them. This is perhaps the most major challenge as staff constantly are striving to deliver the care and feel they have little time for anything else. This is why issues related to change management are so important in helping staff to take note of new or different ways of working to help them meet the competing demands of healthcare today. Within this, the need to use research evidence in practice remains critical.

SUMMARY

This book has, in many ways, given a story of some aspects of research development in healthcare. It has not focused on the 'big' research agenda – that is the numerous major research programmes that are ongoing – rather it has focused on the context in which research developments have been undertaken at local level and a number of efforts to contribute to emerging change. In many respects it gives a snapshot of some developments relating to research in one country at the end of the 20th century. In so doing it has perhaps served to demonstrate the complexity of implementing new ways of working that span, in research terms, from an initial idea for research that needs to be undertaken to situations that, given sufficient evidence, involve changes in healthcare delivery at a local level.

Throughout this text a range of issues have been addressed, from strategic management of research through to personal learning experiences. While it has been noted that the concept of 'getting research into practice' has given way to the notion of evidence-based practice, the simple fact remains that much still needs to be done to help and support healthcare practitioners at all levels to become involved, as appropriate, in knowledge development through research or in utilization of research knowledge in their own clinical area. One of the major challenges in healthcare in the 21st century is for all healthcare practitioners to feel that they can say with confidence that they do use research in their practice.

REFERENCES

Bryar R M, Jose Closs J, Baum G et al 2003 The Yorkshire BARRIERS project: diagnostic analysis of barriers to research utilisation. International Journal of Nursing 40(1): 73–84
Clifford C, Murray S 2001 A pre and post test evaluation of a project designed to facilitate the development of research in practice in a hospital setting. Journal of Advanced Nursing 36(5): 685–695
Clifford C, Murray S, Kelly S 2002 Clinical effectiveness, education and healthcare practitioners. Learning and Teaching in the Professions 1(1): 6–21

Department of Health, Central Office for Research Ethics Committees, http://www.corec.org.uk

Department of Health 1999 Involvement works: second report of standing group of users in NHS research. NHSE/HMSO, London

Department of Health 2000 The NHS plan: a plan for investment: a plan for reform. http://www.nhs.uk/nationalplan [accessed 11 August 2000]

Department of Health 2001 Research governance framework. HMSO, London

European Union (EU) 2001 Directive 2001/20/EC of the European Parliament and the Council of 4 April 2001 on the approximation of the laws, regulations and administration provisions of the member states relating to the implementation of good clinical practice in the conduct of clinical trials on medical product for human use. European Union, Brussels

Higher Education Funding Council for England 2001 Research in nursing and allied health professions: report of task group 3. HEFCE and Department of Health, London

National Research Register (NRR) 2003 Update Software, Oxford, http://www.update-software.com/national/

NICE 2003 London National Institute for Clinical Excellence, http://www.nice.org.uk

Thompson C, McCaughan D, Cullum N, Sheldon T, Thompson D, Mulhall A 2002 Nurses use of research information in clinical decision making: a descriptive and analytic study. University of York. Report presented to the NHS R&D programme in evaluating methods to promote the implementation of R&D. University of York, York

Wilmshurst P 2002 Institutional corruption in medicine. British Medical Journal 325: 1232–1235

Wye L, McClenahan J 2000 Getting better with evidence: experiences of putting research into practice. King's Fund, London

Index